Person-centred Primary Care

Primary care, grounded in the provision of continuous comprehensive person-centred care, is of paramount importance in the delivery of accessible and effective health care around the world. The central notion of person-centred care, however, relies on often-unexamined concepts of self, or understandings of what it means to be a person and an agent. This cutting-edge book explores contemporary pressures on the sense of self for both patient and health professional within a consultation and argues that building new concepts of the self is essential if we are to reinvigorate the central tenets of person-centred primary care.

Contemporary trends such as shared decision-making between health professionals and patients and promoting self-management assume those involved are able to make their own decisions and take action. In practice, however, medicine often opts for reductionist perspectives of patients as passive mechanical systems and diseases as puzzles. At the same time, huge political and organisational changes mean time and resources are scarce, putting further pressure on consultations. This book discusses how we can start to resolve these tensions. The first part considers problems posed by the increasing bureaucratisation of primary care, the impact of information technology in the consultation, the effects of chronic disease on our sense of self and how an emphasis on biology over biography leads to over-diagnosis. The second part proposes solutions based on a strong ontology of consciousness, concepts of creative capacity, coherence and engagement, and will show how these can enhance the self-esteem of patients and doctors and benefit their therapeutic dialogue.

Combining theoretical perspectives from philosophy, sociology and healthcare research with insights drawn from clinical practice, this edited volume is suitable for those researching and studying primary healthcare, communication and relationships in healthcare and the medical humanities.

Christopher Dowrick is Professor of Primary Medical Care at the University of Liverpool, UK.

T0174944

Routledge Advances in the Medical Humanities

www.routledge.com/Routledge-Advances-in-Disability-Studies/book-series/
RADS

New titles

Dementia and Literature
Cross-disciplinary Perspectives
Edited by Tess Maginess

Reading the Psychosomatic in Medical and Popular Culture
Something. Nothing. Everything
Edited by Carol-Ann Farkas

Medicine, Health and the Arts
Approaches to the Medical Humanities
Edited by Victoria Bates, Alan Bleakley and Sam Goodman

Suffering Narratives of Older Adults
A Phenomenological Approach to Serious Illness, Chronic Pain, Recovery and Maternal Care
Mary Beth Morrissey

Medical Humanities and Medical Education
How the Medical Humanities Can Shape Better Doctors
Alan Bleakley

Learning Disability and Inclusion Phobia
Past, Present and Future
C. F. Goodey

Collaborative Arts-based Research for Social Justice
Victoria Foster

Person-centred Health Care
Balancing the Welfare of Clinicians and Patients
Stephen Buetow

Digital Storytelling in Health and Social Policy
Listening to Marginalized Voices
Nicole Matthews and Naomi Sunderland

Bodies and Suffering
Emotions and Relations of Care
Ana Dragojlovic and Alex Broom

Thinking with Metaphors in Medicine
The State of the Art
Alan Bleakley

Forthcoming titles

The Experience of Institutionalisation
Social Exclusion, Stigma and Loss of Identity
Jane Hubert

Person-centred Primary Care

Searching for the Self

Edited by Christopher Dowrick

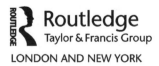

Routledge
Taylor & Francis Group

LONDON AND NEW YORK

First published 2018
by Routledge

2 Park Square, Milton Park, Abingdon, Oxfordshire OX14 4RN
52 Vanderbilt Avenue, New York, NY 10017

Routledge is an imprint of the Taylor & Francis Group, an informa business

First issued in paperback 2019

British Library Cataloguing in Publication Data
A catalogue record for this book is available from the British Library

Library of Congress Cataloging in Publication Data
Names: Dowrick, Christopher, 1951– editor.
Title: Person-centred primary care : searching for the self / edited by
Christopher Dowrick.
Other titles: Routledge advances in the medical humanities.
Description: Abingdon, Oxon ; New York, NY : Routledge, 2018. | Series:
Routledge advances in the medical humanities | Includes bibliographical
references and index.
Identifiers: LCCN 2017032012| ISBN 9781138244184 (hbk) | ISBN
9781315277073 (ebk)
Subjects: | MESH: Patient-Centered Care | Self Efficacy | Resilience,
Psychological | Creativity | United Kingdom
Classification: LCC R727.3 | NLM W 84.7 | DDC 362.1–dc23
LC record available at https://lccn.loc.gov/2017032012

ISBN: 978-1-138-24418-4 (hbk)
ISBN: 978-0-367-88578-6 (pbk)

Typeset in Times New Roman
by Wearset Ltd, Boldon, Tyne and Wear

Contents

Contributors

Christopher Dowrick is Professor of Primary Medical Care, University of Liverpool, and a GP in Liverpool, UK. He is Chair of the WONCA Working Party for Mental Health and Professorial Research Fellow in the University of Melbourne.

Iona Heath is a retired GP and Past President of the Royal College of General Practitioners, London, UK.

Stefan Hjörleifsson is a GP and Associate Professor, Department of Global Public Health and Primary Care, University of Bergen, Norway.

George Hull is Senior Lecturer in Philosophy, University of Cape Town, South Africa.

Sally Hull is Clinical Reader in Primary Care Development, Queen Mary University of London, and a retired GP, London, UK.

Kjersti Lea is Associate Professor, Department of Education, University of Bergen, Norway.

David Misselbrook is Associate Professor of Family Medicine, Royal College of Surgeons in Ireland – Medical University of Bahrain, Kingdom of Bahrain.

Joanne Reeve is Professor of Primary Care Research, Hull-York Medical School, and a GP in Hull, UK. She is past Chair of the Society for Academic Primary Care.

Deborah Swinglehurst is Clinical Reader and NIHR Clinician Scientist, Queen Mary University of London, and a GP in Ipswich, UK.

Preface

Christopher Dowrick

Why primary care needs theories of the self

Primary care, grounded in the provision of continuous comprehensive person-centred care, is of paramount importance in the delivery of accessible and effective health care around the world. Primary health care professionals, including general practitioners and family doctors, are encouraged to work collaboratively with their patients, fostering shared decision-making and promoting self-management. This assumes that patients (and doctors) have agency and capacity, that they have the ability to make their own choices and decisions and the power to take action in a given situation.

But these assumptions are problematic, and there are many factors working against them in contemporary primary care. The huge political and organisational changes which are currently engulfing primary care place intense pressures on the sense of self for both patient and doctor within the consultation.

In this book we will explore these problems and pressures, and offer solutions to them based on explicit theories of the active self. We will argue that the sense of self – for both doctor and patient – is under intense threat, that urgent remedies are needed, and that building new concepts of the self are essential if we are to reinvigorate the central tenets of person-centred primary care.

Our intention is both simple and profound. Our principal motivations in proposing the centrality of the self in primary care are to offer hope to those entering the field, to encourage those jaded by their current experience in practice, and to provide vital underpinning to the generalist cause.

An afternoon surgery

Imagine for a moment that you are a family doctor about to start your surgery on a sunny Monday afternoon. You have had a relaxing weekend. You find you have plenty of energy today, with enough mental space to think about what you are doing, rather than just reacting routinely to the problems your patients present.

The first person you see is 71-year-old Edith Brown, who comes in with her daughter Emma. She has several chronic diseases and is in persistent pain. She has recently been in hospital with a chest infection. The specialists have prescribed her some water tablets to relieve pressure on her heart, but she doesn't want to take them because she won't be able to leave her house for fear of needing the toilet. She feels the hospital doctors didn't listen to her properly, and is worried about losing her independence. You wonder first why Edith didn't explain this to the doctor she saw in the outpatient clinic last week, and then wonder what you should recommend she do about her water tablets. Is her independence more important than her physical health?

Your second patient is Fred, 46 years old and an unemployed single parent of two teenagers. During his previous appointment, two weeks ago, Fred complained of been feeling 'drained'. You asked him to fill out a screening questionnaire to find out if he was depressed, measured his blood pressure, and ordered some blood tests. Today you have to inform him that the results from the questionnaire indicate that he may be depressed, and that the blood tests show that he has developed 'pre-diabetes'. You are uncertain about what to say to Fred. Should you offer him these two new diagnoses and the treatments that would follow from them? Or will doing so just add to the burdens he is already experiencing in his life?

The next person to see you is a woman with gynaecological problems. You offer her a pelvic examination and work out a management plan together, and feel quite comfortable with how the consultation is going. But then you notice on your computer screen a prompt for Recent Smoking Data. Aware of a feeling of slight irritation, you point to the screen and tell her, 'Now my computer's asking me whether you smoke.' You don't really want to discuss this, because it doesn't seem relevant to the consultation, but you feel you ought to mention it as the computer has flagged it up. 'Who is in charge of this consultation?' you grumble to yourself.

Then Millie arrives. She is in her 70s and has lived with her tyrannical mother for many years, until her recent death. Millie has made several appointments to see you while her usual doctor is on sabbatical leave. These consultations have seemed rather rambling and inconsequential to you. If you are being brutally honest with yourself, you have just been trying to keep things ticking over until her regular doctor returns. Today your main aim is to get her out of the door within her allotted ten minutes. Suddenly, Millie gets up out of her chair, turns round, and sits back down on your lap. You are utterly astonished. No patient has ever done this to you before. You realise time is no longer your primary issue, and you will have to start this consultation all over again.

Fortunately your next patient has cancelled. You take the opportunity of a few minutes' break to compose yourself, with a cup of tea and a ginger biscuit.

Mrs. Sayyid, who is in her late 80s, is brought in by her daughter Amal, who tells you she is finding it increasingly difficult to support her mother. Her mother's mild dementia is becoming worse. She repeats the same questions over and over again as she cannot remember the answer. She is distressed that her husband (who has been dead for many years) has 'gone missing'. Amal says 'she isn't herself anymore doctor. It is as if she is the one who is missing.' You reflect on Amal's statement for a moment. Mrs Sayyid is obviously not missing, because you can see her sitting there in front of you. Perhaps Amal means that something essential about her mother, her sense of being a person, has disappeared. Is that something you could – or should – discuss with them in the consultation?

Then Ken breezes in – or rather wheezes in – for one of his regular medication reviews. You have known Ken for a long time. He is 67, used to be a dock worker, and now has severe chronic pulmonary disease. After listening to his chest and checking his lung capacity, you ask him how his health is affecting his life. He reports that he has finally given up cigarettes, but admits that he is still drinking quite a lot of whiskey. You congratulate him on his success with stopping smoking, but then pause for a moment. Should you now bring up the latest health guidance on permitted weekly units of alcohol?

You think you have finished for the day, and are beginning to work your way through the pile of blood tests and other messages that have been accumulating during your surgery. Then your receptionist rings through to tell you that an urgent patient has arrived and asked to see a doctor straightaway. It just says 'very unwell' on your list. Heather walks through the door. She sits down, whispers, 'I feel so ill,' and dissolves into tears. Chastened by your earlier experience with Millie, you mentally put your pile of paperwork to one side, and turn your full attention on the person sat in front of you.

Threats to the self

You will meet these people again, along with several others, as you read through the following chapters. They all illustrate some of the key themes that we discuss throughout the book.

Whether we are doctors or patients, threats to our sense of self are coming from all directions: the effects of suffering on patients' lives, political and organisational changes within primary care, a focus on technology and biology within the consultation, and the implicit assumptions of reductionist scientific paradigms. The work of both doctor and patient becomes increasingly bureaucratic and routinized, as evidence from clinical epidemiology is translated from guidelines into key performance indicators.

Our patients' sense of self can be severely affected by the suffering they experience, whether it be the vitiating impact of the daily grind of socioeconomic deprivation, the fragmenting effects of living with sustained domestic violence, the catastrophic consequences of serious, life-changing disease, or coming face to face with the reality of impending death.

Despite our best efforts to respond to such problems, effective person-centred care is becoming increasingly difficult to practice. The pressures on primary care to comply with a plethora of clinical guidelines and public health agendas, however well-intentioned they may be, all too often conflict with the person-oriented approach which is the hallmark of good general practice encounters. Organisational changes make this more problematic. As practices become bigger the opportunities for continuity of care, for seeing the same doctor on a regular basis, decrease. And in the UK the current general practice workforce crisis, with too few doctors available to meet the needs of our patients, further reduces the possibility of offering the essential personal elements of care. Sally Hull and George Hull argue that general practitioners and their patients, including Edith Brown, suffer from epistemic disadvantage. The current emphases within health care systems on specialist knowledge and bureaucratic approaches lead to situations in which information communicated by the patient is unfairly discounted, and in which GPs don't have the interpretative resources to make sense of their own professional activities.

The primary care consultation, for generations assumed to be the quintessential medium for personal contact between doctor and patient, is now dominated by the presence of technology in the form of the computer. As Deborah Swinglehurst explains in her chapter, the computer brings additional voices into the room, making ever more strident demands for our attention. An increasing proportion of our consultations is conducted remotely, by telephone or other devices. This may help us to meet our access targets but it significantly reduces our opportunities for therapeutic engagement with our patients.

Medical education, whether at undergraduate or vocational training level, has little or nothing to say to us about what it means to be a person, about what might constitute the self. Family doctors fill this vacuum by employing metaphors and explanatory practices derived from a reductionist scientific paradigm. General practice consultation research indicates that we tend to view our patients as passive mechanical systems and their diseases as puzzles, seeing ourselves as problem solvers and controllers of disease. This view may make it simpler for a GP to speed through a busy surgery, but it runs completely counter to our rhetorical public statements about self-care and collaboration. Stefan Hjörleifsson and Kjersti Lea argue that we tend to favour biological over biographical interpretations of the problems of patients like Fred, leading to over-diagnosis and the medicalisation of normal human suffering.

Searching for the self

The solutions for many of these problems lie in socio-economic, political and organisational changes. Problems of poverty, deprivation and abuse cannot be rectified within the consulting room, but demand broader structural approaches. However we consider that recovering a sense of self, for both patients and doctors, is an essential prerequisite for making genuinely person-centred primary care a practical reality (Dowrick *et al.*, 2016).

In the second half of this book we propose a set of theories and concepts on which versions of an active self can be based. We begin by addressing two major problems. The first is socio-political, the advent of totalitarian approaches to health care. The second concerns the physicalist orientation of medical thought. For Iona Heath, the self is the holder of subjective experiences built up over a lifetime, an agent with some ability to shape and influence that experience. The relentless pressures of industrialised medicine threaten the subjectivity of patients like Millie, and of the doctors who seek to care for her. She reminds us that the relief of suffering is at the core of medical practice, and that intersubjective dialogue between doctors and patients is crucial to its achievement. David Misselbrook then presents the contemporary – and often acrimonious – debate between those who see the consciousness of patients such as Mrs. Sayyid as merely a by-product of brain function, and those who see patients and their doctors as moral agents with a degree of free will, moral responsibility and human dignity. He argues for a strong ontology of consciousness, involving full personhood and moral responsibility.

Christopher Dowrick considers the utility of the concept of coherent persons engaged in leading their lives, for example in relation to patients like Ken who are living with long term conditions, and reflects on the notion of embodied selfhood as a basis for understandings the self in more problematic cases such as dementia. He discusses ideas of the social or distributed self, no-self and multiple selves, and indicates how these may provide the basis for concepts of 'shared mind' in the consultation. Finally, Joanne Reeve explains how we can unlock the creative capacity of the self in response to illness. She proposes a model of the Creative Self, powering the work of daily living, balancing resources and demands, with the ability to navigate the flow of daily living. She describes how expert generalists can work with patients like Heather to develop and apply individual management plans to address illness, and argues for bringing back into focus something which has been allowed to slip out of view and into the shadows in recent years.

Processes

In the course of the book we will introduce you to – or remind you of – major contemporary thinkers including Mikhail Bakhtin, Zygmunt Bauman, Havi Carel, David Chalmers, Miranda Fricker, Galen Strawson and Charles Taylor. We will provide a series of vignettes and clinical scenarios, based on genuine but confidentially amended cases, to show how our theories and concepts can enhance the sense of self for patients and doctors alike, and in so doing improve the therapeutic dialogue. We will give a full set of references for each chapter, and offer a glossary of the main technical terms, sociological and philosophical, to be found throughout the book.

While all our chapters stand on their own, they are also connected. In the process of creating this book we have met together at symposia and workshops to discuss our ideas, and we have critically reviewed each other's contributions. Each of our chapters has also been reviewed by at least two external peer-reviewers.

You will find recurring themes, including concepts of personal agency and ideas based on virtue ethics; concerns about pressures and constraints on the primary consultation, and arguments about the balance between biology and biography, or between systems and persons. You will also find some areas of disagreement between us, particularly when we are each seeking to describe what we mean by the self. For some of us it is slippery, elusive and intangible; for others it is more clearly delineated and apparent.

This is not a worry for us. We do not wish to establish the truth of selfhood, whatever that mercurial entity might be. Our desire is rather to encourage reflection, discussion and debate about the self as a critical concept for primary healthcare; a concept that we believe to be at serious risk of extinction, in danger of vanishing completely from view.

Reference

Dowrick, C., Heath, I., Hjörleifsson, S., Misselbrook, D., May, C., Reeve, J., Swinglehurst, D. and Toon, P. (2016). Recovering the self: a manifesto for primary care. *British Journal of General Practice*, 66 (652): 582–583.

Acknowledgements

We are grateful to the following people for their comments on and reviews of various elements of this book:

Josie Billington, Barry Dainton, Philip Davis, Anna Dowrick, Ronald Epstein, Don Hill [now deceased], James Hawkins, Anna Luise Kirkengen, George Lewith [now deceased], Anne MacFarlane, Carl May, Catie Nagel, Lara Nixon, Becky Rawlinson, Jane Roberts, Joachim Sturmberg, Liz Sturgiss and Peter Toon.

1 Recovering general practice from epistemic disadvantage

Sally Hull with George Hull

What is the role of the general practitioner?

Though a visit to the GP is a familiar part of life for most of us, the question, 'What does a GP do?' can be hard to answer.

In particular, it is harder to answer than the equivalent question asked about – for example – an anaesthetist or a hepatologist. Each of these has a well-defined area of specialist knowledge and core skills. Equally, each has a clear set of hurdles to negotiate in the achievement of specialist status.

By contrast, the GP is a generalist. In spite of evidence of the importance of general practice for population health within health systems, there have been repeated assaults on the value of the generalist's role (RCGP, 2012; Starfield *et al.*, 2005). So it is worth pausing to consider some distinctive aspects of the work of a GP.

Although generalists may work in many settings the term, particularly in the UK, usually applies to the contemporary GP. A frequent formulation is that GPs work at the interface between illness and disease and between individual health and population health, a place where serious disease has low prevalence, where diagnostic tests are less precise and where a diagnostic formulation involves judgement and is always risky (Heath and Sweeney, 2005). For our purposes, what is important is that the role of the GP is to be at the interface between illness and disease. In other words, the GP must co-ordinate biomedical knowledge and expertise with the subjective experience of the patient in their consulting room. As Heath and Sweeney put it, the GP must bridge the gulf between the 'map of medical practice' and the 'territory of a patient's suffering'. Iona Heath discusses this dilemma further in her chapter later in this book.

The general practitioner stands in a distinctive type of relation to their patients, not replicated in specialist medicine. This is lucidly captured by Ian McWhinney:

> The commitment of a GP is to a person, not to a person with 'a limited list' of diseases. If GPs are to fulfil their place it is important that their commitment is unconditional. We cannot say I will be your doctor as long as you are not housebound, dying, or have a complicated condition in which I don't

have much expertise. The unconditional nature of the commitment means that the relationship between GP and patient is open ended.

(McWhinney, 1981)

A number of things can flow from this relationship. It allows intimacy and friendship to grow, based on a mutual interest in the patients' health, and at its best the relationship is one of trust, which is both precious and very fragile.

The everyday work of co-ordinating biomedical knowledge with the subjective experience of patients is made up of a mass of *situated judgements*. And it is vital that a GP's judgement calls be informed by the psychosocial context of the patient as much as they are by biomedical expertise. A GP's situated judgements are supported by the findings of medical science and are often improved by computer-based decision aids. However, these decisions remain hedged about with uncertainty. Is it right to stick to the hypertension guideline for this elderly lady? How best to incorporate my knowledge about the risks of polypharmacy alongside her expressed desire not to take any more medicines?

The skilled practice of generalist medicine may include knowing a set of abstracted rules and recommendations. But the work of a skilled GP could not be substituted by the mechanical application of a list of rules – however long. This is because it relies crucially on making situated judgements with the patient. Decisions are rooted in the immediacy of patient context. The capacity to make such judgements is continually refined and reinforced as the practice of individual GPs is reviewed in the social context of the professional group.

We should consequently understand a skilled GP not as someone who has learned a set of rules and guidelines and applies them automatically, but primarily as someone who has acquired and maintains a number of settled dispositions of character which give rise to perceptive context-sensitive judgements as they interact with patients. Another way of making this point is to say that the expert GP has acquired and manifests a distinctive set of *virtues*.

The concept *virtue* is most familiar from moral theory. In applying it to medical practice it is important to avoid misunderstandings.

Theorists in the field of philosophical ethics disagree about what constitutes a morally good individual. The *deontological* approach says the morally good individual is the individual who knowingly conforms in their behaviour to rule-like norms including duties and obligations. The *consequentialist* approach says the morally good individual is the individual whose actions maximise some valued outcome (such as pleasure). *Virtue ethics*, in contrast, says the morally good individual is the individual who possesses certain settled dispositions of character: the *moral virtues*, including honesty, courage, generosity, and others. The dispositions of character highlighted by virtue ethics form the basis for characteristic patterns of perception and behaviour.

In claiming that successful medical training to become a general practitioner involves the acquisition of a set of virtues, we are not claiming that becoming a skilled GP is the same thing as becoming a morally good person. Whilst it is plausible that possession of certain moral virtues is a necessary condition of true excellence in general practice – a point we will come back to later in this chapter – possessing the moral virtues alone is clearly not sufficient to make someone an excellent GP.

The claim being made here is about form rather than content. The *form* of (much of) the expertise possessed by an excellent GP is comparable to the form of the moral expertise possessed by a morally good person.

The *content* of the virtues which best serve the practice of medicine will vary between its different branches. The development of virtue requires a consciously reflective approach, supported by structures which encourage and 'envirtue' participants (Toon, 1999).

Discussing moral virtue, John McDowell writes:

> If one attempted to reduce one's conception of what virtue requires to a set of rules, then, however subtle and thoughtful one was in drawing up the code, cases would inevitably turn up in which a mechanical application of the rules would strike one as wrong – and not necessarily because one had changed one's mind; rather, one's mind on the matter was not susceptible of capture in any universal formula.
>
> (McDowell, 1998)

Similarly, David Wiggins argues that acquiring a moral virtue is a matter of acquiring a capacity of 'moral or practical perception', which he also describes as 'a high order of situational appreciation'. Here he is making a point which he takes to extend to practical matters beyond the domain of morality:

> From the nature of the case the subject matter of the practical is indefinite and unforeseeable, and any supposed principle would have an indefinite number of exceptions. To understand what such exceptions would be and what makes them exceptions would be to understand something not reducible to rules or principles.
>
> (Wiggins, 1998)

A virtue is an acquired disposition, so a good generalist medical training should develop settled dispositions of character in a GP which enable them to make the right judgements in consultation with their patients. One of the goals of training must be to ensure these distinctive virtues are explicit, and become second nature to GPs.

Of course rules and guidance are useful, but they are not a substitute for *'the educated improvisations of a virtuous ... perceptual sensitivity'* (Fricker, 2007).

In sum, GPs are generalists whose medical expertise consists, to a significant degree, in the possession of a set of virtues. These virtues enable the GP to develop an on-going doctor-patient relationship constructively and make situated medical judgements about a patient informed both by biomedical knowledge and psychosocial information.

This chapter seeks to contribute to an understanding of general practice in medicine, and propose ways in which it can be strengthened. It draws on recent work in critical social theory, which has focused on the importance of how we – as society and as individuals – relate to persons *in their capacity as knowers*. Philosophical work following this epistemic direction in social theory has emphasised the centrality of developing one's capacities as a producer and conveyor of knowledge, and how this contributes to the development of a flourishing individual life. It has also drawn attention to types of wrongful harm which individuals can suffer at the hands of society in their capacity as knowers.

Our focus is on the roles of doctors and patients as knowers in a well-functioning health service. It principally considers two aspects of the role of knower:

- the *testimonial*: the doctor and patient as people who convey knowledge to others;
- the *hermeneutical*: the doctor and patient as people who are able to make sense of their own experiences and activities, and whose experiences and activities are comprehensible to other salient role-players.

This chapter highlights two forces or trends which, we will argue, have adversely affected general practice – and thereby the good functioning of the UK health service – by providing GPs with deficient or distortive explanatory resources with which to frame their professional activity. These two forces or trends are:

- the *specialist paradigm*: a privileging of specialist medicine as more skilled, more serious, more worthy of attention and funding, and more deserving of high status than generalist medicine;
- the *bureaucratic paradigm*: a trend towards managing medical activities at all levels in the health service by seeking to identify and maximise discrete quantifiable unit outputs – whether tonsillectomies, root canal procedures, or ten-minute consultations.

Specifically, the chapter makes three claims. First, both the specialist paradigm and the bureaucratic paradigm have made GPs, and GPs-in-training, less able than other medical practitioners to understand the nature of their medical activities and experiences associated with them, thereby making them less well equipped to perform their role excellently. Relative to the medical community, GPs have suffered a *hermeneutical disadvantage*. Second, important among the skills or virtues that GPs must acquire and manifest are epistemic virtues, which enable them to build doctor-patient relationships over time, in ways which respond constructively to the communicative efforts of patients. Third, when GPs are put at a hermeneutical disadvantage relative to the medical profession as a whole, this makes them less able to appreciate, and thus develop, the skills – including epistemic virtues – which they need in order to provide an excellent service to patients.

We also argue that GPs in the UK, reflective about their practice, have sought to fill in the gaps in their training, thereby improving the theory and practice of their profession. Such efforts require institutional encouragement if the UK health service is to have a well-functioning generalist service in the long term.

The marginalisation of general practice

Not long after the National Health Service was founded, a trend towards privileging hospital-based medicine within Britain's public health sector began to emerge.

Although specialist medical practice in the UK had begun to grow from the mid-nineteenth century – spurred on by urbanisation and market competition – it was only after the foundation of the NHS that sub-specialism really took off (Rivett, 1986). This specialism was almost exclusively located in hospital settings and was linked to the rise of the single disease model and the rapid advances in technology which transformed hospital practice. Importantly, increased technology-driven specialism resonated with the public self-image of the times, summed up in the phrase 'white heat of technology'.

> The Britain that is going to be forged in the white heat of this revolution will be no place for restrictive practices or for outdated methods.
>
> (Wilson, 1963)

These various strands contributed to what we can call the *specialist paradigm* in British medicine from the mid-twentieth century onwards.

Generalist medicine was out of tune with the spirit of the time, and in this period the threats to general practice came from a pervasive neglect. This included a material neglect of physical resources such as buildings, staff and equipment. Alongside this general practice was affected by an attitude of disrespect from other branches of medicine. Relatedly, while the specialist paradigm thrived, there was a vacuity of theorising about the discipline of general practice and its potential contributions to population health (Collings, 1950). The pervasive view within medicine and within broader society during this period is summed up in the words of Lord Moran, an influential post-war president of the Royal College of Physicians, who declared that GPs were merely the doctors who 'fell off the ladder', lacking the 'outstanding merit' to become top hospital specialists.

It is important to note that this hostility towards general practice was neither new, nor confined to the UK. Joanna Brooks (2016) used data from the oral history collection in the USA National Library of Medicine to chart the trends in disparagement of primary care in American medical schools between 1936 and 1985.

Even before medical school training began the new recruits came across messages at university interviews about what was to be avoided:

> Clearly, if you mentioned the word 'general practitioner,' you had said something terribly wrong. He asked me, he said, 'Well, what kind of physician do

you want to be?' And I said, 'A general practitioner.' And he spent the next 20 minutes berating me, and telling me that I could go to a GP school if I wanted to, but [school name] produced specialists, and was a cut above that kind of interest.

(Paediatrics, Tufts University School of Medicine 1964)

Alongside the overt cultural hostility to general practice came messages that being intelligent and professional were incompatible with choosing primary care. This builds a powerful conceptual framework, a shorthand of stereotypical ideas, prejudices and feelings, that becomes synonymous with the idea that choosing general practice is a failure. Obstacles to any change in these attitudes were perpetuated by the underrepresentation of primary care faculty members in training settings. This decreased the opportunities for role models and mentors, and meant that the unwritten curriculum of the primacy of specialist medicine became embedded in the hierarchical power structures of medical education and the early years of practice.

The specialist paradigm in medicine led to neglect of, and prejudice against, generalist medicine. This not only led to material neglect of general practice and relative disrespect for GPs. It also had important epistemic consequences for GPs which this chapter will explore further in due course. In particular it meant that GPs were not equipped through their training to make full sense of their role, activities and experiences in the health service. With no opportunity to illuminate the work of generalists there was an absence of experience and associated theory, which emptied out the perception of this branch of medicine for all but the most determined of students.

It's hard, because there's no way to know what general internal medicine is, on the basis of a medical residency in a hospital. It just ain't there. I mean, there's no overlap, all the things you do as a medical resident, while it gives you a lot of knowledge and certain skills, has very little to do with the real life of a practicing internist which is overwhelming with outpatients. Now a surgeon, I think, he's learning in the hospital what he's going to be doing. He's doing what he's going to do. The internist doesn't.

(Internal medicine, Northwestern University School of Medicine 1947)

The hostility and denigration described here from historical data in the USA has not disappeared either from medical schools or from the current environment of medical practice in the UK.

In 2016 the British Journal of General Practice ran an editorial in which academics based in General Practice and Psychiatry wrote about 'Not such friendly banter' describing the continuing denigration of these two specialties (Baker *et al.*, 2016). Such lack of credibility and status has widespread consequences for recruitment, posing a threat to the health service and ultimately to the health of patients.

The point is reiterated by Val Wass in the 2016 report on future careers in general practice:

One of the most commonly heard anecdotes in medical schools is the description of the packed lecture theatre in the first week. The lecturer asks the students, 'How many of you want to become general practitioners?' Only three raise their hands, enabling the lecturer to comment disparagingly, 'Well tough, half of you will "end up" as GPs.'

(Wass and Gregory, 2017)

Whilst there is good evidence that early clinical exposure to general practice, including authentic and positive role models, is important in promoting it as a positive career choice, there still remains a problem of finding the language to encompass the territory.

the GP tutor we had she was an absolutely amazing GP, because I saw from her that you can … because there is a saying, isn't there, that it is easy to do the job badly, but it's hard to do it well as a GP.

(Nicholson *et al.*, 2016)

Although this quote includes the sense that the student intuitively recognises the well done job of this GP tutor, there is also in that phrase 'I saw from her that you can … because' once again, the difficulty of articulating the elements of this excellence. This imbalance of interpretive resource-for-articulation between generalist and specialist settings contributes to a reluctance of students to take up general practice. It contributes to the relative poverty of explanatory theory applied to the everyday work of general practitioners.

This poverty of theoretical resources for general practice is a theme we will take up again when we discuss ways in which general practice is subject to hermeneutical disadvantage. Before that, however, we must introduce the notion of epistemic disadvantage.

What is epistemic disadvantage?

How can somebody be harmed or disadvantaged by society specifically in their capacity as a knower?

The most obvious answer would probably concentrate on practices of withholding knowledge from people or deliberately providing them with misinformation. Alternatively, one might point to the inequitable patterns of access to knowledge through education in a country like the UK.

However, recent work in critical social theory has identified further, less obvious, ways in which the power dynamics of a society can disadvantage people specifically as knowers. Particularly relevant for reflecting on the position of general practice within the British health service are two types of epistemic harm identified by Miranda Fricker in her book *Epistemic Injustice* (2007).

In her work, Fricker focuses primarily on the epistemic disadvantages which people of particular gender, sexual-orientation and racialized groups can suffer when there is pervasive prejudice against them in society. But the types of epistemic disadvantage which she identifies have wider application. Fricker's principal focus is on cases of epistemic disadvantage which constitute *social injustice*: cases of relative epistemic deprivation on the part of certain groups which mean they have been wronged socially and have a legitimate grievance. However, the types of epistemic disadvantage she discusses may also manifest in ways which, though they have significant effects, do not count as social injustice.

Fricker identifies two important forms of what she calls epistemic injustice. The first is *testimonial injustice*, which occurs when an individual or group suffers a deficit in credibility due to prejudice. An example of this would be when a society does not allow the testimony of black people as much weight in court as that of white people, due to pervasive racial prejudice in a society. A less institutional example would be when people are less inclined to believe what women say about political issues than they are to believe what men say, due to pervasive condescending stereotypes about women. In both these examples, people are harmed in their capacity as conveyors of knowledge because of the existing social prejudice against them. Testimonial injustice describes the ways in which we may routinely and unfairly dismiss claims to knowledge from those people who are not sufficiently like ourselves, or hold a low position in an established social hierarchy.

The second form of epistemic injustice is *hermeneutical injustice*. This exists due to the fact that people rely on a collective stock of conceptual and discursive resources in order to make their social experiences intelligible both to themselves and to others. The shape which that stock of interpretative resources takes will be determined in no small part by prevailing power relations within society. When one group in a society is relatively marginalised and thus excluded from the processes by which collective hermeneutical resources are generated, this may have an adverse impact on the ability of members of that group to make their social experiences intelligible.

Fricker discusses the example of a society in which women are hermeneutically marginalised. In such a society a woman who suffers sexual harassment may find nothing in a society's collective hermeneutical resource which is adequate for the articulation of her experience. She may find that the existing hermeneutical resources 'have a lacuna where the name of a distinctive social experience should be' or alternatively she may only find a concept that distorts her experience. It is no coincidence that in a society where men disproportionately occupy positions of power in the generation of discourse – in the media, in academia, in government – little effort will be put into developing forms of discourse adequate to the experiences of sexual harassment which women specifically are subject to. In such a situation it may be neither of interest to, nor in the interests of, the men in positions of power to devote attention to developing such a discourse. But beyond that, men who have not experienced the kinds of sexual harassment which women are subjected to may not be in a position to initiate the process of building a vocabulary and forms of discourse to delineate the subject.

Testimonial disadvantage in general practice

Earlier we described how the rise of the specialist paradigm in British medicine led to a pervasive depiction of GPs as second-rate medical professionals. It was suggested at the start of the chapter that this is an incorrect and unfair characterisation of GPs, who have a crucial and distinctive role to play at the interface between illness and disease – a role which requires a distinctive set of virtues. Thus within the medical community GPs are the subject of a degree of unfair prejudice.

Testimonial disadvantage affecting GPs

Given the hierarchy which the specialist paradigm entrenched in British medicine, it should not come as a surprise if GPs experience testimonial disadvantage in their interactions with other medical professionals – if the testimony of GPs is dismissed due to an unfair prevailing prejudice. Indeed, within the sphere of the medical community, we should not be surprised if GPs suffer *testimonial injustice*. But the hierarchical presumptions of the specialist paradigm did not only remain within the medical community, they also seeped out into broader society to some extent. Hence at times GPs may find themselves at a testimonial disadvantage in their interactions with patients.

To say that GPs suffer testimonial disadvantage relative to specialist medical doctors is not to say that they are subject to a social injustice. GPs are among the most materially privileged members of society, and their status as educated middle-class doctors ensures that they tend to have far more credibility than most members of society. Even within the medical community, they have higher status and greater power than many other professionals – such as nurses and midwives.

Nonetheless, it is worth making the point that GPs are subject to testimonial disadvantage relative to medical specialists because of the harmful impact this can have on others – specifically, on their patients. The following case illustrates how this is not only frustrating for GPs but potentially harmful to patient care.

Consider the example of 71-year-old Edith Brown, who is burdened with several chronic diseases and persistent pain. She has just come home from hospital after an admission for a chest infection. As her GP you visit her, to find her daughter Emma, who lives some miles away, is present – with concerns that her mum has been dizzy and is becoming frailer. Hospital specialists have stressed the importance of extending her medication list to include two further antihypertensive agents, and she has an upcoming out-patient appointment to check on compliance with the regime. In spite of your expertise in generalist medicine, your experience in managing multimorbidity and the adverse effects of medication, and your appreciation of how Edith is affected in her daily life by her symptoms, it may well be the case that in the eyes of the patient and family you suffer from a credibility deficit. Your medical knowledge is seen as neither deep nor specialised, in comparison with the hospital specialist – and indeed your own training may have reinforced these ideas. Together these factors may work against the best interests of your patient.

Testimonial disadvantage affecting patients

If patients can be harmed indirectly by the credibility deficit of GPs relative to specialist doctors, they can also be harmed directly due to the credibility deficit they themselves suffer.

Doctors are by no means immune to prejudice. Given the central importance of co-ordinating between biomedical knowledge and the subjective experience of illness in their work, it is crucial for GPs to be aware of ways in which their own prejudice can distort their interactions with patients. Both general societal prejudices and prejudices specific to the medical profession can conspire to create an unwarranted credibility deficit on the part of a patient. Such testimonial disadvantage adversely affects patients both in their capacity as knowers and because it can lead to unsatisfactory clinical outcomes.

Consider the case of Edith Brown again.

Since her recent hospital admission for a chest infection, two months ago, Edith has hardly gone out of the house. Previously she had enjoyed her volunteering sessions in a local charity shop. Her daughter Emma brings her to the surgery and explains that her Mum has been to outpatients and they are very happy with her blood pressure, but she is concerned that she has lost some independence. Edith says:

'They told me to keep taking the water tablets ... to strengthen my heart. It was difficult to say what I wanted to ... and that I didn't choose to take them. I know they are trying their best to help, but I don't want to be a burden like this.'

Medical practice is replete with stories about failures of communication. Here we focus on the epistemic dimension of these encounters – situations where patients suffer a disadvantage in their capacity as an informant with a claim to knowledge, the patient as a person with knowledge about their condition.

In this situation Edith Brown has an essential contribution to make to the encounter which is based on her personal experience of living with the illnesses she has, and with the multiple medications she has been given. But there is a problem. In the pressured experience of the outpatient department (or a hurried contact in a GP surgery) she has difficulty in voicing her experience, and in addition has only a hazy conception of the construct which we can refer to as the effect of polypharmacy, but which she may see as the kindly expert attempting to solve each of her medical problems. Hence it is difficult to voice the choice based on her knowledge, which comes from living with her symptoms, that she would prefer to be biomedically speaking sicker, but psychosocially conceived better and still able to get to the charity shop without the inconvenience caused by the diuretic. Too often she may be reduced to silent acquiescence.

Patient stories are rarely expressed in standard medical discourse and can easily be assigned a deflated epistemic status. The hearer may refuse to concede that certain forms of information – such as the detailed narrative of the illness experience – are relevant to the task in hand. This excludes certain types of knowledge from either informing current practice, or from contributing to reform of these practices:

> I've only got ten minutes, patients give a lot of irrelevant stuff. I have to hone in (*sic*) on what's important.
>
> (Kidd and Carel, 2016)

Even a sympathetic clinician may fail to see the full value of a story. GPs, like other doctors, may develop a prejudice against acknowledging the relevance of patient testimony which is not framed in scientific medical terms. The current emphasis on the biomedical description of disease can exacerbate this problem, with less attention paid to the subjective experience of being ill. This is reinforced by the structure of contemporary healthcare where work is increasingly task-based rather than patient-focused, and limits the opportunities for establishing sustained patient contact which in turn can foster the recognition of patients' epistemic contribution to their care. This privileging of a certain type of content, vocabulary and procedure can lead to relevant patient testimony being discounted, and can diminish the doctor's ability to take properly informed decisions. Here the prejudices of the GP due to their training, and the everyday structures and task-based routines of contemporary healthcare, are responsible for testimonial disadvantage suffered by the patient.

These experiences are detrimental to the patient by undermining their ability and willingness to take part in further interpersonal exchanges. The person will gradually lose their epistemic confidence as they endure the constant erosion of their credibility, which over time crushes their confidence in their epistemic capabilities. People in this situation will not expect what they say to be heard, and in time may not speak at all.

As well as the possibility of testimonial disadvantage which is specific to a medical encounter, people who are ill are also vulnerable to becoming the subject of testimonial injustice derived from the prevalent negative stereotypes of illness within society. Being physically unwell, and dependent on others for help, additionally places the patient in a position of vulnerability which erodes social and epistemic confidence and capacities during an encounter. Chronically sick people are a group liable to be regarded as less credible by society in general, particularly when they are also elderly and/or poor. Doctors are not immune to pervasive social prejudice, and those same prejudices in the doctor's mind and sensibility can very well lead them to discount or not take seriously the testimony of a patient in consultation.

Fricker (2007) emphasises that such stereotypes and prejudices typically operate: 'without any focussed awareness' and are 'culpably resistant to the evidence', and thus irrational.

Such stereotypes may include a connotation of incapacity, diminished agency, psychological fragility and social vulnerability. A broad theme of such stereotypes is of the body's condition as an expression of morality, and the fact of illness is often conceived as a mark of moral, social or epistemic failure (Carel and Kidd, 2014).

At the beginning of this chapter it was proposed that a GP's expertise consists to an important degree in the acquisition and maintenance of a set of virtues. Due to the possibilities of testimonial injustice in their interaction with patients described here we may conclude that one of these virtues is what Fricker calls 'the virtue of testimonial justice'.

Though Fricker suggests it is a moral virtue that all people should aim to cultivate, we suggest that it is of particular importance for GPs, as testimonial disadvantaging of patients in their interactions with a GP is particularly likely to lead to adverse consequences. The virtue of testimonial justice involves a settled disposition of character making an individual critically aware and perceptive of possibilities of distortion by prejudice of the testimony of a person they are interacting with. Developing the virtue of testimonial justice for GPs involves developing reflective awareness of ways in which what a patient says and how they say it, can lead them to discount or distort the patient's testimony. Only in this way can they develop the consistent ability to adjust for and correct this tendency on their part.

Hermeneutical disadvantage in general practice

In this section we propose that the hierarchy within medicine normalised by the specialist paradigm has given rise to a situation in which GPs are hermeneutically disadvantaged relative to other medical professionals. In addition, we propose that some of the recent history of general practice in the UK can be understood as the actions taken by GPs to overcome the hermeneutical disadvantage they have faced.

The examples of hermeneutical disadvantage which Fricker (2007) considers in *Epistemic Injustice* involve groups which are marginalised relative to society as a whole, such that they do not take part in the construction of mainstream hermeneutical resources for self-interpretation and thus may find themselves unable adequately to conceptualise or communicate important aspects of their social experience. For example, if women are hermeneutically marginalised, they may find there is no term or style of discourse adequate to capture the experience of sexual harassment; if homosexual people are hermeneutically marginalised, they may find the only style of discourse available to capture their experiences is distortive and pathologising.

The claims in this section about GPs are much more modest. GPs are not hermeneutically marginalised relative to society as a whole. Rather, their participation in the propagation, and to some extent the formulation, of medical discourse gives them a hermeneutically privileged position – and many GPs contribute to knowledge production and public discourse in fora beyond their professional sphere. What hermeneutical disadvantage GPs are subject to does not amount to social injustice, and the impression that GPs are somehow victims is certainly to be avoided.

However, the denigration of general practice in medical schools and the lack of GPs as teachers and leaders in those fora as a consequence of the specialist paradigm during the twentieth century meant that a discourse specific to general practice and adequate to the experiences and challenges facing GPs was to a large extent lacking in Britain. If general practice was defined at all, it was defined in terms of what it was not.

David Morrell joined a practice in 1957, soon after the foundation of the NHS, and describes his early experience as follows:

> The early weeks and months in the consulting room were confusing, and I was filled with feelings of guilt. The knowledge and skills acquired in hospital just did not seem relevant to the many problems I encountered, and when a proper hospital type patient presented, there was never time to carry out the type of examination that I had learnt in hospital posts.
>
> General practitioners responded to this situation in different ways. Some became desperate and depressed at the demands being made on them, which differed so much from their expectations and training. They complained: 'This is not the medicine for which we were trained.'
>
> (Morrell, 1998)

This piece, along with the earlier quoted passages about training for general practice in medical schools in the USA, illustrate the hermeneutic gaps and the confusing spaces which mark out the lack of a conceptual framework at the heart of general practice.

As Fricker says:

> relations of unequal power can skew shared hermeneutical resources so that the powerful tend to have appropriate understandings of their experiences ready to draw on as they make sense of their social experience, whereas the less powerful ... have at best ill fitting meanings to draw on in the effort to render them intelligible.
>
> (Fricker, 2007)

Unable to draw on a mainstream medical discourse about the types of interaction GPs needed, and the distinctive skills and virtues required of them, British GPs found themselves in a disorientating situation.

The long-term solution for such a situation of hermeneutical disadvantage must involve a shift in power and representation, with more GPs providing senior leadership in medical schools and a shift in attitudes about general practice. Meantime a group of people who find themselves hermeneutically marginalised can make some progress in overcoming hermeneutical disadvantage by coming together and, in the company of others who also find that the mainstream discourse is dissonant with their lived experience, starting to mint a new vocabulary and discourse which are adequate to their professional experience.

For comparison, here is what Miranda Fricker writes about 'the mechanism of consciousness raising' through 'speak-outs' in the history of the women's movement:

> Put a number of people together who have felt a certain dissonance about an area of social experience, and factor in that each of them will have a different profile of immunity and susceptibility to different authoritative discourses, and it is not surprising that the sense of dissonance can increase and become critically emboldened.

(Fricker, 2007)

Sometimes, Fricker writes, during such speak-outs 'the hermeneutical darkness … suddenly lifted' on areas of women's experience such as 'post-natal depression' and 'sexual harassment', which had been obscure to them due to a structural prejudice in the collective hermeneutical resources working to their disadvantage.

In the case of GPs in the UK who were hermeneutically marginalised relative to the medical profession, in the face of these common experiences, there were a number of responses which produced a body of theory and engaged practice which has lasted until recent times. Much of this work emerged from energetic activism within general practice. It was often from the crucible of small group work among GPs, and a few interested outsiders, that productive innovation and change emerged. One instructive example of this was the work done in Balint groups.

When Michael Balint started his groups for GPs in the 1950s his explicit aim was to provide some training for GPs in the techniques of psychotherapy to be applied to the many cases in which physical symptoms were brought to the doctor, but the problem was most likely a psychological one. He reported as follows:

> It is generally agreed that at least one quarter of the work of the general practitioner consists of psychotherapy pure and simple. Some investigators put the figure at 50% or even higher; but the fact remains that the present medical training does not properly equip the practitioner for at least one quarter of the work he will have to do.

(Balint, 1954)

This approach brought the external, and at that time, powerful, discipline of psychotherapy up against the untutored world of general practice. The expectation was that GPs could learn to use psychotherapy techniques to attend properly to 'the other part of medicine' (Balint, 1961).

However, as Balint worked with GPs over a period of years leading seminar groups, the idea of foisting a specialist service into the consulting room gradually gave way to the provision of a meeting place between GPs and psychoanalysts for the study of the everyday work of general practice.

By the 1970s the foreword to *Six minutes for the patient* was able to identify the primacy of the consultation in general practice, albeit with a wry glance at the continuing professional denigration from specialists and from GPs themselves:

> this book is first and foremost an account of the ordinary consultation, the sort in which GPs are engaged thirty or forty times each working day. This is what we were looking at – or it might be truer to say looking down on initially.
>
> (Balint and Norell, 1973)

One of the ideas brought from psychotherapy was that aspects of relationships which may be problematic for the patient could be reflected in the relationship with their doctor. With the change in paradigm brought about by this shift in gaze from the patient and disease to the doctor-patient in relationship, many aspects of the work of general practice were brought into view which previously had been unobserved, remained out of sight, and certainly not thought to be worth serious study (Hull, 2003).

Much of the case material for these groups came from longstanding, troubled or stuck relationships with patients. Within the group doctors were encouraged to listen and observe, not to be tied down by theory, whether brought from psychoanalysis or from the medical school, but to retain the discipline of both identifying with the patient and then standing back and testing out an observation in dialogue. Sometimes this can lead to an intense, intimate contact. In the short, but repeated, consultations of general practice this can give a freedom to some patients to use the doctor in the way that they choose, and frees the doctor from the primary task of trying to discover why the patient talks, feels and behaves in this way. The patient in due course will be able to provide the answers.

Many of the aphorisms that became part of the common culture of general practice emerged from these seminars: the idea of 'the drug doctor' and the various ways this can be used in diagnosis and therapy, the continuing relationship and deepening intimacy with a patient builds up 'a mutual investment company' which both parties can draw on and the 'collusion of anonymity' which can occur when multiple specialists have seen, treated and discharged the patient, when many doctors are involved but no one appears responsible for taking decisions.

The ideas which started in these seminars have had an influence far beyond the groups of doctors who attended, and helped to construct core working theories for general practice by recognising the central role of the consultation and the requirement for teaching about general practice as an independent discipline. GPs gained the confidence to look critically at both the organisation and the content of their work. They also recognised that it was not the problems that were brought to them in clinical encounters in the surgery which were wrong, but the educational framework devised in hospitals which was not fit for the job. The work in groups also brought to mind that to provide effective care it is important to look beyond the demands of the immediate encounter with the patient (Tudor Hart, 1988).

As well as providing a safe environment in which GPs could discover, or re-fashion, concepts to capture previously hidden or inadequately articulated aspects of practice, such groups continue to be places where the development of the necessary virtues-for-practice can be supported.

Developing vocabularies and discourses in which to frame the experiences and challenges which GPs face is of benefit to GPs. But – arguably more impor-tantly – it is also of benefit to their patients, because it allows practising GPs to build a set of resources which they can use to improve their professional prac-tice. In this chapter we have already seen one example of a specific area where it would help GPs to achieve an articulated and reflective awareness: in the cultiva-tion and maintenance of the virtue of testimonial justice. There are doubtless many other examples.

Digital health: consumer convenience or constructed inarticulacy?

As general practitioners develop vocabulary and discourse to articulate the dis-tinctive virtues manifested by GPs in doctor-patient encounters, and substantiate the value of such relationships for the health service, this may prove important in resisting developments which may have adverse consequences for patients.

This point can be illustrated with an example taken from a modern digital encounter. This is not to deny the profoundly enabling contributions of digital access to health information, and its emerging contribution to possible solutions to the problem of matching demand and access.

Let's consider this scenario:

Carol is a salaried GP working at a surgery which has started offering web based consultations for a limited range of clinical problems. That morning she is alloc-ated one for 'elbow pain' from a patient who has been seen once or twice over the past two years by his regular GP.

The form involves several computer screens of confirming demographic information and then a series of answers to clinically focused, closed questions, from which Carol gathers that for the last six weeks he has had a pain on the outside of the elbow which is worse on picking things up.

He reports no other symptoms. Carol is confident this is a case of tennis elbow, and is able to send him a link to a YouTube video of eccentric exercises for lateral epicondylitis and an information leaflet. She signs off the e-mail encounter sug-gesting that if his pain hasn't improved in 4–6 weeks he rings the open access physiotherapy service for further advice.

Compare this:

Mohammed Aziz is on my surgery list that morning. It's a good morning for me, alert and refreshed with an unfilled slot in my session. As I call him in I am unusually alert to seeing that he wears a suit, worn but pressed. As he sits my imagination races away as I notice the unfilled shoulders of his jacket and how he sits or indeed shrinks into the seat with an attitude which speaks of resignation. I ask what I can do for him, and he explains the details of his painful elbow, that he works in a restaurant and that repetitive work with the cooking pans must be the cause of his pains. He falls silent with a slight frown, which is clearly asking to be taken further. As I examine his arm I try out a comment about whether he has lost some weight. And then he tells me about leaving his accountancy business in Pakistan, and that his wife and family are not yet with him, and that although living with a relative he is lonely, getting home too late for family meals. I take a minute to show him how to do the eccentric exercises for his epicondylitis, touching his scrawny arm in a gesture of solidarity, and suggest he sees our social prescribing co-ordinator, who may have ideas about alternative work or other opportunities for him.

This was a consultation which gave satisfaction to the doctor as well as some relief to the patient. The doctor was able to use technical medical skills as a bridge to move from an instrumental role in providing a plan for his painful elbow, into a relational role in seeing and hearing his distress and disappointment in the direction his life has taken, and accepting the role of witness to his predicament. The arm pain and his life course are inextricably linked, and the doctor can engage – at the patients' pace – in rebuilding a painful narrative.

The web-based consultation demands a different type of work from doctors and patients (Casey *et al.*, 2017). The process of taking a history has been devolved back to the patient, and inherent in this process is the Procrustean bed which fits the patient's story into one of 100 standard scripts. The GP is disburdened from the relational work done during a consultation, and it becomes a solely transactional matter. Now all of this can happen during a face to face consultation, but it would appear that by using this device, which digitally embodies biophysical notions of technical efficiency, the patient is being denied access to the relational content of the consultation. In turn this may model a progressive narrowing of the shared interpretative enterprise, in which narratives are built and reinforced by doctor and patient which acknowledge the links between the biological, psychological and social aspects of life.

Recent challenges to practice

The decades leading up to the 1990s were a period of medical dominance and self-regulation, but the 1990s brought new challenges.

These challenges came from the application of a scientific-bureaucratic model of medical care – scientific in the sense of relying substantially on biomedical knowledge, and bureaucratic in the sense of relying on rule-based implementation: 'One way best' of doing things, a 'single answer' to any given clinical problem. The rise of scientific-bureaucratic medicine reflects an exercise of social power in the form of managerial control: we can call this the *bureaucratic paradigm*.

Indeed it has been argued that the change in the model of medicine can be linked to a change in social relations. The earlier 'personalised/bedside' model was associated with the dominance of the patient over the physician. In contrast the more abstracted hospital based biomedical model made the perspective of the patient marginal to doctors' decisions about diagnosis and treatment (Harrison, 2009).

The traditional relationship with a patient has characteristics of indeterminacy. For example medical care is co-produced and emerges over time, it includes the physician's reaction to the patient's account and the patient's response to the physician's diagnosis and advice.

The managerial project within medicine aims to gain control over this process. It requires the conceptual commodification of the outputs of medical care. The basic strategy of commodification is to establish a classification system into which unique cases can be grouped in order to provide a definition of medical output or workload. Good examples of these commodified outputs include the Health Care Resource Group (HRG) within the hospital system, and the Quality and Outcomes Framework (QOF) within primary care. Harrison goes on to assert that the biomedical model of medicine is conceptually aligned with managerial views of the world with key assumptions in common – in particular a view of medical pathology which can be abstracted from the individual patient. It is then consistent with a population-based conception of medicine in which individuals with the same disease should be treated the same way, that cases within a category are fundamentally homogeneous.

Within general practice this is seen in the trend towards stratifying activity into product lines to improve access and efficiency. Organisational efficiency is a laudable aim, but a primary focus on access and segmentation also subtly introduces new conventions that describe 'how things are'. This subordination of clinical content to market segmentation appears progressive – and indeed necessary – in the face of resource constraint, but it can be particularly troubling in primary health care which is replete with exceptions and surprises and the resistance of people refusing to conform to the textbook case or become reduced to formulaic rules and protocols.

The process of commodification then starts to become normalised – and even internalised. Hence GPs may see QOF performance as the key measure of quality in practice, and may participate in restructuring practice to enable the unbundling by management of product lines within a corporate structure.

This 'crowding out' of the tacit knowledge which medicine employs, but which cannot be codified, may initiate a major change in doctors' views of their medical selves. First the idea that the technical/industrial elements of medicine which have become much more prominent are thus the most important; second that corporate medical care leads to the transformation of the doctor patient relationship into the necessary efficiency of a series of isolated encounters.

This creates a cultural dissonance between the professional institutions of general practice, which continue to espouse a biopsychosocial model of medicine whose concern is with the social and psychological context of the whole 'situated' patient, and the apparatus of medical research and institutional payment which is largely predicated on a narrow approach to the biomedical model. For practising GPs the espousal of holistic medicine can become merely rhetorical, or at worst contribute to the sense – once again – that they are acting in an unsympathetic context with tools that do not suit their task as conceived. These ideas are developed further in the next chapter by Stefan Hjørleifsson and Kjersti Lea.

The suggestion here is that the application of social power through the model of scientific bureaucratic medicine has altered the conception of what it is to be a doctor – especially a general practitioner. In its place is an isolated encounter based approach with an emphasis on transactional solutions to bite-sized biomedical symptoms. The process has loosened and dismantled the interpretative social understanding which is embodied in the tacit knowledge and practice identified with being a good doctor. Such a process is also visible in aspects of the manifestation of digital encounters, as detailed in the previous section and discussed further in Deborah Swinglehurst's contribution.

The bureaucratic paradigm, like the specialist paradigm, creates a risk that general practitioners will be in a position of hermeneutical disadvantage. However it does so in a different way to the specialist paradigm. The specialist paradigm left – to a large extent – a gap where the mainstream discursive resources for GPs' self-understanding should have been: it portrayed GPs simply as *not specialist doctors*, indeed as *failed specialists*. What the bureaucratic paradigm does is something different. It provides GPs with discursive resources to understand their role, the challenges they face, and the behaviour required of them. But it speaks to the GP in the language of the assembly line, dividing the work of the GP into discrete homogeneous quantifiable tasks. It thus provides the GP with a self-understanding which is distortive – since it leaves out the uniqueness and unpredictability of the personal interaction in a one-to-one consultation, the challenges which come with it, and the virtues needed to negotiate them. Consequently the bureaucratic paradigm, no less than the specialist paradigm, is likely to leave the GP somewhat disorientated in their day-to-day work – but in this case it is a disorientation arising from a dissonance between how the mainstream discursive resources available to them portray their work, and the lived experience of that work itself.

Resistance and renewal

The social context for most health care within the UK remains the NHS, still widely valued as an institution which practises redistributive social justice on a daily basis:

The collective principle asserts that … no society can legitimately call itself civilised if a sick person is denied medical aid because of lack of means.

(Bevan, 1952)

The importance of the role of generalism in health systems is supported by a body of work largely collected by Barbara Starfield (2003). She provides evidence that a strong generalist presence within medicine is associated with better health outcomes, a more equitable distribution of health in populations and that it reduces and even protects patients from inappropriate specialist care. However, this evidence is frequently offset by a resistance which is embedded in cultural norms and existing power structures.

In 2016 Chand Nagpaul, chair of the BMA's GP committee, was moved to write testimony to the continuing unease that GPs have with the nature of their own profession. This at a period when, despite the calls for more generalism, the numbers of doctors in the UK going into general practice is falling, and the relative resource for primary care has shrunk.

He notes that one of the most frustrating questions for GPs about their occupation is: 'What do you specialise in?' 'Reply that you are a GP, and you will be met with the reaction that you have somehow not achieved your full potential or that 'proper doctors' all specialise in something'. For Nagpaul, such a response indicates a fundamental lack of understanding that being a GP is a speciality in its own right. Indeed, he argues, 'being a caring and competent GP demonstrates the greatest of medical accomplishments'. He goes on to state that there is a formal call for general practice to be recognised as a specialty in its own right and that 'We hope that this will be the first major step in rectifying this prejudicial status' (Nagpaul, 2016).

The fact is that after 70 years of general practice within the health service the GP committee of the BMA is still calling for the role of general practice to be equally recognised within the body of medicine. This complaint goes beyond the unequal shares of resource that come to general practice – important as this is. Instead the emphasis here is on the relationship of general practice to the specialisms within medicine. It is important to recognise the role of non-economic factors which contribute to this problem. A redistribution of resources, including educational resources, towards general practice will not solve this on its own. Disrespect and prejudice remain important factors which maintain and perpetuate the current hostility which contributes to the failure of marginalised disciplines within medicine to flourish.

Renewal comes from many sources, often unexpected. One of several examples is the recent focus on multi-morbidity, including research by academics with experience of general practice in socially deprived areas (Barnett *et al.*, 2012). Conceptually alien to specialism, this emergent focus on complexity in practice presents us with an insistent demand that it lies at the heart of everyday general practice:

Although complexity is under-represented in the research literature, it is common place in general medical practice, where the challenges are 'horizontal', integrating not only at the level of the clinical encounter, but also in the co-ordination of services to support patients with multiple problems. The challenge of carrying out research on multimorbidity is to reflect, investigate, inform and improve these aspects of generalist clinical practice.

(Mercer *et al.*, 2009)

This powerful organising principle has a range of associated ideas which engage in a similar space, concepts such as polypharmacy and the burdens and harms of overtreatment.

We have argued that the role of the general practitioners is valuable and distinctive within medicine. The GP's position at the interface between the patient's experience of illness and the biomedical conceptualisation of disease demands distinctive virtues, and its own body of terms and discursive resources to help the reflective GP orientate themselves in practice. Important among these, we have argued, is the virtue of testimonial justice, which GPs must cultivate and maintain if they are to be adequately responsive to the patient's story in their medical judgements. GPs' ability to orientate themselves and achieve a constructive professional self-understanding has been undermined by prevailing power relations and governing ideas within medicine in the UK. Both the specialist paradigm and the bureaucratic paradigm have – in their different ways – put GPs in a position of hermeneutical disadvantage.

But the history of British general practice provides hope, and demonstrates how GPs have, from the ground up worked to fill in the discursive gaps and correct the discursive distortions regarding their medical activity. Such reflective processes need to find support and resonance from the work of front line GPs, so that the self-understanding of general practice continues to be effectively renewed.

Key learning points

1   Generalism within medicine is simultaneously disparaged within the body of medicine, but also recognised as an essential means of ensuring an efficient and equitable provision of medical service within a society.
2   This prejudicial situation leads to a situation of hermeneutical injustice, in which there is an absence of collective self-interpretative resources for the accurate delineation of the generalist sphere and its future development.
3   Epistemic disadvantage in the form of testimonial disadvantage – prejudicial to the unique situated knowledge of being a person with a disease – remains commonplace within medicine.
4   A key professional virtue for GPs to cultivate is that of testimonial justice, which enables them to resist unfairly discounting or dismissing information coming from the patient due to prejudice.
5   Both the specialist paradigm and the bureaucratic paradigm have undermined GPs in their professional activity to a significant degree. Both engender inadequate discursive resources with which to make sense of their

practice or provide distortive discursive resources which are dissonant with the lived experience of general practice. Such forms of epistemic disadvantage affect recruitment into generalist careers.

6   Historically resistance and renewal have emerged as practitioners engage with each other and with patients within the current social context, to build the ideas, and broadly speaking the hermeneutical resource needed for the future.

References

Baker, M., Wessely, S. and Openshaw, D. 2016. Not such friendly banter? GPs and psychiatrists against the systematic denigration of their specialties. *British Journal of General Practice*, 66 (651): 508–9.

Balint, M. 1954. Training general practitioners in psychotherapy. *British Medical Journal*, 1 (4854): 115–20.

Balint, M. 1961. The other part of medicine. *Lancet*, 1: 40–2.

Balint, E., Norell, J.S. 1973. *Six minutes for the patient: interactions in general practice consultation.* London: Tavistock.

Barnett, K., Mercer, S.W., Norbury, M., Watt, G., Wyke, S. and Guthrie, B. 2012. Epidemiology of multimorbidity and implications for health care, research, and medical education: a cross-sectional study. *Lancet*, 380 (9836): 37–43.

Bevan, A. 1952. *In Place of Fear*. London: Simon and Schuster.

Brooks, J.V. 2016. Hostility During Training: Historical Roots of Primary Care Disparagement. *Annals of Family Medicine*, 14 (5): 446–52.

Carel, H. and Kidd, I.J. 2014. Epistemic injustice in healthcare: a philosophical analysis. *Medicine Health Care and Philosophy*, 17: 529–40.

Casey, M., Shaw, S. and Swinglehurst, D. 2017. Online consultation systems: case study of experiences in one early adopter site. *British Journal of General Practice*, in press.

Collings, J. 1950. General practice in England today. *Lancet*, 1: 555–85.

Fricker, M. 2007. *Epistemic Injustice: Power and the Ethics of Knowing.* Oxford: OUP.

Harrison, S. 2009. Co-optation, commodification and the medical model. *Public Administration*, 87: 184–97.

Heath, I. and Sweeney, K. 2005. Medical generalists: connecting the map and the territory. *British Medical Journal*, 331: 1462–4.

Hull, S.A. 2003. *The study of the doctor patient relationship.* In Lakhani, M. (ed.) *A celebration of general practice.* Oxford: Radcliffe.

Kidd, I.J. and Carel, H. 2017. Epistemic injustice and illness. *Journal of Applied Philosophy*, 34: 172–90.

McDowell, J. 1998. *Virtue and Reason* in *Mind, Value and Reality.* Cambridge Mass: Harvard University Press.

McWhinney, I. 1981. *Family Medicine.* Oxford: OUP.

Mercer, S.W., Smith, S.M., Wyke, S., O'Dowd, T. and Watt, G.C. 2009. Multimorbidity in primary care: developing the research agenda. *Family Practice*, 26 (2): 79–80.

Morrell, D. 1998. As I recall. *British Medical Journal*, 317 (7150): 40–5.

Nagpaul, C. 2016. *Recognising our work as a specialty.* Available at: http://bma-mail.org.uk/JVX-4F1DY-9E36IEOQ88/cr.aspx

Nicholson, S., Hastings, A.M. and McKinley, R.K. 2016. Influences on students' career decisions concerning general practice: a focus group study. *British Journal of General Practice*, 66 (651): 768–75.

Rivett, G. 1986. *The development of the London hospital system 1823–1982.* London; King Edward's Hospital Fund of London.

Royal College of General Practitioners (RCGP) 2012. *Medical Generalism: why expertise in whole person medicine matters.* London: RCGP.

Starfield, B. 2003. *The effectiveness of primary care.* In Lakhani, M. (eds) *A celebration of general practice.* Oxford: Radcliffe.

Starfield, B., Shi, L. and Macinko, J. 2005. Contribution of primary care to health systems and health. *Milbank Quarterly*, 83: 457–502.

Toon, P. 1999. *Towards a philosophy of General Practice: a study of the virtuous practitioner.* Occasional Paper 78. London: RCGP.

Tudor Hart, J. 1988. *A new kind of doctor: the general practitioner's part in the health of the community.* London: Merlin Press.

Wass, V. and Gregory, S. 2017. Not 'just' a GP: a call for action. *British Journal of General Practice*, 67 (657): 148–9.

Wiggins, D. 1998. *Needs, values, truth.* Oxford: Clarendon Press.

Wilson, H. 1963. *'Labour's plan for science'.* Speech made at the Annual Labour Party Conference, Scarborough.

2 Mismanagement in general practice

Stefán Hjörleifsson and Kjersti Lea

Introduction

General practice is currently in a problematic position where the biomedical model increasingly becomes the organising principle for care, while the range of health problems that general practitioners deal with only lends itself to a limited extent to management in terms of this same model. Too often, this leads to clinical mismanagement and failure, not least when patients present with problems caused by social disadvantage, trauma and loss of meaning, when they have problems that practitioners perceive as 'medically unexplained', and in the management of 'risk'.

Medical practice relies on a set of presuppositions about its subject matter and goals, and the relevant types of knowledge and skills to apply to the subject matter in order to reach these goals. Usually, discussions about these presuppositions are not part of practice. Even in debates about medical practice, healthcare organisation and research, this shared set of presuppositions often goes unnoticed or undebated.

One can start to gain an understanding of the importance of the underlying presuppositions of medical practice from British sociologist Nicholas Jewson. In 1976 he introduced the concept of 'cosmology' to describe the underlying presuppositions of the field. According to Jewson, medical cosmologies are the ways of thinking that define a professional field and unite its practitioners:

> They are conceptual structures which constitute the frame of reference within which all questions are posed and all answers are offered. Such intellectual gestalt provide those sets of axioms and assumptions which guide the interests, perceptions, and cognitive processes of medical investigators…. [c]osmologies are not only ways of seeing, but also ways of not seeing. Cosmologies prescribe the visible and the invisible, the imaginable and the inconceivable. They exclude in the same moment as they include.
>
> (Jewson, 1976, pp. 225–6)

On Jewson's account, the dominant cosmology of medicine has changed radically in modern times. Medicine has turned away from being person-oriented towards an object-oriented cosmology. Beginning in the nineteenth century, medical practitioners came to rely less on observing the patient at the bedside and more on specialised examinations, the findings of posthumous pathological examinations and, eventually, surgical procedures. Accordingly, disease as conceived at the level of organs and tissues became the object matter of medicine. Subsequently laboratory measurements and visualisations provided an access to the disease even further removed from the thinking, feeling person who is the patient. Other scholars, extending this analysis, have also traced its philosophical and methodological origins to Descartes' ideas about the inanimate and researchable body (Leder, 2013). With a different concept, one can say that the movement away from the subjective experience of the patient towards objective entities seen in the laboratory or at autopsy means that the 'philosophical anthropology' of medicine undergoes a fundamental change. The underlying, philosophical understanding of what man (*anthropos*) is as the object matter of medicine is at the heart of the cosmology of medicine. Within the object-oriented cosmology, the philosophical anthropology of medicine is that of the human body as an object that can be researched and manipulated.

Another concept that describes many of the same presuppositions of medicine as Jewson sought to capture is that of the 'biomedical model'. Since its introduction by George L. Engel in 1976, the concept of the biomedical model has been used in various ways to encompass the dominant presuppositions of medical research and practice. As David Misselbrook argues in Chapter 5 of this book, in the biomedical model the object matter of medicine is the body devoid of subjective experience. This view of man, as a philosophical anthropology of medicine, is reductionist, and implies a mind-body dualism. In Engel's words,

> [the] dominant model of disease today is biomedical, with molecular biology its basic scientific discipline. It assumes disease to be fully accounted for by deviations from the norm of measurable biological (somatic) variables. It leaves no room within its framework for the social, psychological, and behavioral dimensions of illness. The biomedical model not only requires that disease be dealt with as an entity independent of social behavior, it also demands that behavioral aberrations be explained on the basis of disordered somatic (biochemical or neurophysiological) processes. Thus the biomedical model embraces both reductionism, the philosophic view that complex phenomena are ultimately derived from a single primary principle, and mind-body dualism, the doctrine that separates the mental from the somatic. Here the reductionistic primary principle is physicalistic; that is, it assumes that the language of chemistry and physics will ultimately suffice to explain biological phenomena. From the reductionist viewpoint, the only conceptual tools available to characterize and experimental tools to study biological systems are physical in nature.
>
> (Engel, 1977)

Since the biomedical model or the objectivist cosmology came to dominate medical practice, the scope of medical practice has been much extended. While the practice of medicine previously was directed towards those seeking help due to accidents or disease, the ambition of medicine gradually has also come to include prevention and early detection and treatment of disease, based on detailed regimes of observation and behavioural instructions for the population.

The French historian-philosopher Michel Foucault provided an early analysis of a broad societal development towards controlling citizens through extensive surveillance, linking this idea to Jeremy Bentham's vision of the 'panopticon' (Foucault, 1997). The panopticon was a prison consisting of a circular building with cells along the external wall, each facing toward a central rotunda which served as the guards' station, from whence the guards could keep all inmates under constant surveillance. Although the guards could not observe all the prisoners at the same time, the latter could not know exactly when they were observed by the guards and thus would at all times behave as though they actually were being observed. In Bentham's view, this was a way of making the inmates effectively control their own behaviour, and thus a 'new mode of obtaining power of mind over mind' which would among other things 'preserve health' and 'invigorate industry' (Bentham, 1995). Foucault observes that, much as inmates in the prison conceived by Bentham, citizens of today must assume that they are constantly under surveillance, and this leads the population to conform by the internalisation of this reality.

The British physician and sociologist David Armstrong has described how, gradually during the twentieth century, the realm of medicine came to include surveillance. Large-scale observations, numerical registration and statistical analyses of entire populations are now used for the purpose of identifying and treating disease at its early stages or even to prevent disease altogether by addressing 'risk factors' and modifying behaviour. According to Armstrong, the rise of surveillance involves a radical extension of the scope of medicine:

> Hospital Medicine was only concerned with the ill patient in whom a lesion might be identified, but a cardinal feature of Surveillance Medicine is its targeting of everyone. Surveillance Medicine requires the dissolution of the distinct clinical categories of healthy and ill.
>
> (Armstrong, 1995, p. 395)

As surveillance, prediction and pre-emptive control becomes the new ideal, the object matter of medicine changes correspondingly. Now medicine deals with all citizens, whose role it is to undergo regular measurements in order to judge their health status, their risk of future illness, and to follow particular rules of behaviour intended to prevent them from falling ill. As defined within the cosmology of medical surveillance we all have a moral duty to subject ourselves to surveillance and to take precautionary actions based on expert interpretations of their risk of disease. The requirement for strict adherence to quantitative measurement and standardised preventive behaviour implies that the subjective perspective of the patient or the citizen is not of interest. Thus, although the scope of medicine in the cosmology of surveillance is more extensive than in the

object-oriented cosmology, both share the feature that their philosophical anthropology is that of patients without regard for their experiences and subjective
points of view.

We now need to turn our attention to general practice and to scholars who
have argued for a worldview – cosmology – or model that is different from the
biomedical model. In the paper from 1977 that includes the description of the
biomedical model we quoted above, Engel made the claim that the biomedical
model needed to be replaced by what he called the 'biopsychosocial model'.
Although a psychiatrist by training and writing primarily about the failures of
the biomedical model within his own specialty, Engel launched the biopsychosocial model as an alternative intended for medicine in general. Another highly
influential author was Ian McWhinney, who in 1978 introduced the person
centred clinical method, suggesting that this was an appropriate method for
primary care medicine: 'Family medicine does not separate disease from person,
or person from environment' (McWhinney and Freeman, 2009).

Since Engel and McWhinney, methods for working with patients as persons
have been developed and disseminated in general practice, mainly under head-
ings such as the patient-centred clinical method (Stewart *et al.*, 2013). The relationship between this method and the biomedical model has also been debated.
Iona Heath and others have suggested that primary care and hospital medicine
are mutually dependent on each other, and that it is necessary for each to be
radically different from the other. In her 2011 Harveian Oration with the title
'Divided we fail', Heath makes a strong argument that it is to everyone's benefit
that general practice operates from its own worldview. She highlights the ability
of general practitioners to remain 'close to their patients and communities and
… observe the generation and progression of illness and disease within particular
life contexts and stories' (Heath, 2011, p. 576). It is this ability that enables
general practitioners to judge who among their patients are likely to benefit from
the investigations and treatment that the hospital specialists with their biomedical science can provide. Without the person-centred services of general practitioners, relying on a cosmology different from that of biomedical science,
hospital specialists would be serving patients beyond their remit. Conversely,
Heath also argues, the limits of the person-centred capacities of general practitioners are such, that if hospital specialists were not available to treat patients
when requested by general practitioners, many patients would receive
insufficient care.

One could thus assume that the current state of affairs is as it should be. A
fundamental division of labour between general practitioners and hospital specialists is in place, and the success of this division of labour hinges on an essential difference between the cosmologies and corresponding methodologies of
general practice and hospitals.

However, these assumptions may not necessarily hold true. There are currently many indications that the biomedical and surveillance model are strongly
influential in general practice. General practice education has little to say about
what it means to be a person or a self. Beyond a general 'patient-centred' or

'person-centred' rhetoric, and communication techniques intended to enable the provision of such care, the notion of the 'self' or the 'person' at its core is rarely unpacked, and neither conceptual nor institutional conditions for providing such care are established. As Deborah Swinglehurst and Iona Heath argue in subsequent chapters, disease-focused clinical guidelines, public health agendas focusing on single diseases and individuals, structured and interventionist electronic records, and expanding medical technologies leave little room for personal interaction between general practitioners and their patients. Bigger practices, workforce shortage and differentiation, and prioritisation of access reduce personal continuity of care.

This has harmful consequences for many patients in general practice, not least for those with complex problems and multimorbidity, those presenting due to problems related to disadvantage or loss of meaning and belonging, and to patients with 'unexplained' symptoms and 'patients' who are without symptoms but 'at risk'. Too often one-sided reductionist and biological approaches trump biographical interpretations of patients' problems, rendering the latter invisible or their relevance inconceivable, leading to harmful overdiagnosis and medicalisation of human suffering. Increased surveillance and registration, with lowered diagnostic thresholds and increased pressure to identify and take action against all pathology at its very beginning, create more patients and more tasks for doctors – tasks that, when defined primarily within the biomedical framework, carry large costs while their benefits are often limited.

As the biomedical model holds a hegemonic position, its limitations invisible and any alternatives inconceivable, it is difficult to express concerns or criticism. One reason for this may be that the presuppositions of the biomedical model have strong footholds in contemporary culture – far beyond the healthcare services.

The biomedical model overlaps with widely shared presuppositions about human nature in our times. According to the Canadian philosopher Charles Taylor, the philosophical anthropology of medicine relates strongly to general cultural assumptions about what human beings are, and the ways of thinking and acting that are suitable for dealing with such beings. These assumptions, according to Taylor, are seldom questioned or systematically debated. In *The ethics of authenticity* (1992), Taylor speaks of a troubling 'inarticulacy' of prevailing moral and ontological intuitions about human nature. This inarticulacy has come to threaten the achievements of modernity, giving free reign to the 'runaway extensions of technological reason' in modern health care (Taylor, 1995).

It seems to us plausible to suggest that different criticisms of modern health care in general, and general practice in particular, coalesce around problems deriving from 'runaway extensions of technological reason'. Taking our inspiration from Taylor and from Drew Leder, whom we will introduce properly below, we suggest that 'inarticulacy' may be a major reason for this, since it implies a lack of engagement with underlying presuppositions of medical practice.

Any practice is grounded on certain values that constitute its framework. These values may be more or less explicit. In times of challenge, conflict or crisis, one is forced to reflect on and perhaps articulate the assumptions and judgments that inform the practice. As Taylor explains, to articulate means to

> try to spell out what it is that we presuppose when we judge that a certain form of life is truly worthwhile, or place our dignity in a certain achievement or status, or define our moral obligations in a certain manner [and thus], we find ourselves articulating inter alia what I have been calling ... 'frameworks'.
>
> (Taylor, 1989, p. 26)

The empowering force of articulation, then, is that it makes clear what is at stake and what the values of the practice are. This makes it possible, and sometimes necessary, for those involved in the practice to take a stand.

If the fundamental values of general practice were clarified, it would be easier to discuss and judge what these values could and should mean for the way such practice is conducted. This seems to be exactly what Drew Leder suggests when he states that 'the 'metaphysics' of medicine must be examined and critiqued, before focusing exclusively on its manifestations' (Leder, 2013, p. 3, Introduction). Furthermore, even when the presuppositions implied in the biomedical model have been analysed and criticised as in Engel's work quoted above, there remains the equally important task of establishing an alternative philosophical anthropology that is theoretically adequate and practically robust enough to counter the dominating position of the biomedical model.

The self and the act of interpretation

It is to the latter task we will now turn. We will seek to establish from philosophical theory basic elements of what it means to be a person. To be able to say anything about what the notion of personhood may imply in general practice, we need an understanding of what being a person generally implies. This is a challenge that Christopher Dowrick also addresses in Chapter 6. In search for such an understanding, we again turn to Taylor who is among the philosophers who have explored the meaning and implications of personhood (Abbey, 2004; Taylor, 1989). Our aim is to sketch an alternative model for medical practice. We hope to indicate how a different philosophical anthropology may contribute to establishing a more adequate and ethically sustainable model for medicine, and specifically for general practice.

According to Taylor, man is a being with a sense of self (Lea, 2015, p. 94; Taylor, 1995). In his elaboration of this claim, Taylor particularly emphasises articulation, morality, sociality, temporality, intentionality and meaningfulness as fundamental to the sense of having a self. As Taylor points out, as humans we express ourselves, we relate to each other, and we ascribe meaning to everything we perceive. Such meaning, Taylor claims, can never be neutral or objective. Meaning is situated and impregnated with values; it is directed by our previous experiences and gives direction to our future (Taylor, 1989, 1995).

Thereby, '[s]elfhood and the good ... turn out to be inextricably intertwined terms', Taylor observes (1989, p. 3). Furthermore, our sense of self is not static. On the contrary, my sense of myself is of a being who is growing and becoming (Taylor, 1989, p. 50), and thus it constantly needs to be revised, or re-interpreted (Lea, 2015, p. 97). This is in short what leads Taylor to assert that man is the 'self-interpreting animal' (Taylor, 1985).

Taylor believes that human beings interpret their lives in narrative terms. When interpreting our lives as an unfolding story, we ascribe meaning to the past and give direction to the future (Abbey, 2004, pp. 38–9; Taylor, 1989, pp. 47, 50–2). This means that as self-interpreters we are also self-narrators (Smith, 2004). For, according to Taylor's view, to be a self 'an individual must locate herself and her action within a larger narrative context; and at least part of what it means to be a self or agent is to engage in (implicit or explicit) acts of self-interpretation and/or 'account-giving' (Baynes, 2010, p. 449). Since our understanding of ourselves thus is regarded constitutive of who we are (Fossland and Grimen, 2001, p. 65), much may be learned about individuals' self-understanding and, in fact, also about who they actually are by studying their narratives about themselves. From this point of view, the stories we tell about ourselves are important and highly relevant to understanding individuals as persons, as well as the nature of the human condition.

In Taylor's own words,

> [s]elf-understanding is constitutive of what we are, what we do, what we feel. Understanding ourselves as agents is not in the first place a theory; it is an essential part of our practice. It is inescapably involved in our function-ing as human beings.
>
> (Taylor, 1985, p. 202)

Thus 'to ask what a person is, in abstraction from his or her self-interpretations, is to ask a fundamentally misguided question, one to which there couldn't in principle be an answer' (Taylor, 1989, p. 34).

On the other hand, an agent's sense of who he is also is fundamentally dependent on his surroundings; on the dominating ideas in his time and his culture, as well as on other people's views and direct response to him, his actions and utterances. In Taylor's words, 'a self only exists among other selves' (Taylor, 1985, p. 35). He holds that the self is dialogical, and that a person's understanding of himself is shaped by how he is seen by and relates to others (Abbey, 2014). Man may in Taylor's view thus be regarded a fundamentally social animal. Consequently, context matters also when we deal with individuals and try to understand them.

Embodiment

We can now take one a further step in direction of philosophical anthropology of medicine. If man is a self-interpreting animal, we now need to establish the contents of the act of interpretation that Taylor claims human beings continuously engage in. What are the sources of human experience? Here we turn to the phenomenological philosophy of Maurice Merleau-Ponty, whose point of departure is that all experience is embodied: 'Human beings are in the world as bodies' (Merleau-Ponty, 1962). There are no human beings without a body, and everything about human beings relates to the fact that they are embodied. The body is a permanent condition of everything we experience; it is the site whence we know the world. Human beings are embodied selves. Everything the self experiences is experienced through and in the body.

It seems to us that to serve as an adequate philosophical anthropology for medicine, a theory of personhood such as Taylor's needs to be firmly linked to a theory of the self as an embodied entity, such as Merleau-Ponty's. The relationship between the self and its body is not contingent or external. The body is not as an impersonal object or a lifeless machine, but an incarnated subject. Or rather, the fact that the body can be regarded as an object of manipulation needs to be supplemented by the perspective that our bodies are the source and origin of all perception and action. The body has a dual existence; it is both an object and a subject.

Taking inspiration from Merleau-Ponty, physician and philosopher Drew Leder has investigated how 'medical theory and practice might be transformed by attending more fully to lived embodiment' (Leder, 1984, p. 34). According to Leder, the notion of the lived body 'leads us toward a medicine of the "intertwining": one that moves back and forth between the physiological and existential dimensions of illness, understanding them as equally significant and mutually implicatory' (Leder, 2013, p. 7, Introduction). From this perspective, the body is not just any material object, but also an 'intending' entity (Leder, 2013, p. 25). The notion of intentionality is paramount to Leder, meaning to be 'bound up with, and directed toward, an experienced world. It is a being in relationship to that which is other: other people, other things, an environment' (Leder, 2013, p. 25). Thus, the notion of the lived body is meant to surpass the mind-body dualism.

Implications

According to Leder, a main corollary of postulating that medical practice is an interpersonal endeavour between embodied subjects, the patient and the practitioner, is that clinical work is interpretive in its nature. Moreover, by

> acknowledging the interpretive nature of clinical understanding, we leave behind the dream of pure objectivity. Where there is interpretation there is subjectivity, ambiguity, room for disagreement. The personal and provisional character of clinical judgment cannot be expunged.
>
> (Leder, 1990a)

In general practice, clinical judgement always has a 'provisional character'. Accepting the interpretive nature of such judgement can perhaps enable us to come to terms with the uncertainty that is inherent in general practice.

If clinical work is interpretive, and if general practice needs a philosophical anthropology inhabited by persons who are embodied selves rather than carriers of objective pathologies, we now need to attend to the status of biomedical knowledge. The question is what status the theoretical models and practical tools of biomedicine can be accorded if the biomedical model, or the objectivist cosmology, is not adequate for the needs of general practice. Here, Leder's concept of 'intertwining' between 'the physiological and existential dimensions of illness' can be of help. Other theoreticians have also sought to envision knowledge practices that combine the explanatory approach of the sciences with the understanding of the humanistic or hermeneutic disciplines. Thus, according to Ricoeur,

> [T]he moment of understanding is characterized by an intuitive, overall insight into what is in question ... marked by a commitment on the part of the knowing subject. The moment of explanation, on the other hand, is marked by the predominance of analysis, the subordination of the particular case to rules, laws, or structures, and by the setting at a distance of the object under study in relation to an independent subject. What was most important, to me, was not to separate understanding from explanation or vice versa.... Interpretation, for me, consists precisely in the alternating of the phases of understanding and those of explanation.
>
> (Ricoeur, 2013, p. 9)

As we explore below, patients and medical practitioners often end up in trouble because they fail to realise that the problems they are dealing with require alternating or intertwining. In the paper *Clinical interpretation*, Leder describes this problem of 'hermeneutical false consciousness':

> [M]odern medicine, I would contend, has been bewitched by a quite different ideal – that of achieving a purified objectivity. Interpretation necessarily implies the existence of subjectivity, ambiguity, opacity. In trying to overcome these bars to absolute knowledge, medicine has sought to escape its hermeneutical foundations and reconstitute itself as a pure science.
>
> (Leder, 1990a, p. 19)

Case stories

We now turn to case stories that we will analyse in light of the above. However, we first much explain their sources, and to emphasise that none of the cases reveals the identity of any real persons. On the one hand, the stories are authentic in the sense that they are synthesised from clinical experience in general practice in Norway over 15 years, from discussions with general practice colleagues in Iceland, Norway and England, including general practice trainee groups in Norway, and from discussions with medical students in Iceland and Norway. The stories thus convey authentic observations of our own and those of many colleagues. On the other hand, no single patient is the source of any of these case stories. Rather, we have extracted, summarised and combined from the above sources.

The context where we have collected most of this material is one where general practice has long held a strong position within a publicly funded health-care system, and general practice is either free at point of entry (England), or patients pay a fee of approximately £18 or €20 (Norway) for each consultation with their general practitioner.

Case one: Zac, who keeps account of his own body

Zac works at a university college. He is 42 years' old, happily married with two children. It is very important for Zac to be physically active, and he spends a fair amount of his time on training. His favourite form of exercise is running, but he also likes to swim, to bike, and to ski. He is on the university college's football team, and he enjoys the occasional tennis match with his friends.

Zac's wife sometimes complains that his training scheme is so engrossing that there is very little time left for her and the children or for him to take his fair share of housework and other practical tasks. In response to this, Zac usually points out that good health is more important than most things and that training is a necessary part of a healthy lifestyle. Besides, Zac would not fancy being a plump, shapeless couch potato, he tells his wife. He wants to be active and fit!

This winter Zac has been bothered with pain in his forearms, so much that it has affected his training programme. This troubles him a great deal, so he decided to see his general practitioner about the problem. The GP referred Zac for physio-therapy. After four treatments, his forearms are starting to feel better. However, Zac is facing a new problem; he has become aware of a painful sensation in his left shoulder that seems to get worse from his swimming sessions. Sometimes the pain in his shoulder radiates towards the neck. Zac is getting anxious that it could trigger the headaches that sometimes are a cause of much frustration to him. He wonders whether he ought to keep a diary of the symptoms in his shoulder and in his arm to check whether he can detect a pattern that may connect the headaches to these problems. It would be quite a nuisance if his headaches were to interfere with his training scheme, as this would prevent him from reaching his personal goal for his next triathlon, so Zac really wants to keep them under control. From his heartrate monitor, Zac can see that the recent training sessions have been less effi-cient than he likes to admit. Perhaps he ought to bring his heartrate readings and the headache diary he is already keeping to his general practitioner.

When Zac hands his doctor the latest documents regarding his pulse rate and head-aches, the general practitioner does not really want to examine them closely. 'What-ever do I know about heartrate variability and triathlon training schedules?' she thinks to herself. 'And in a sense, what do I really care?' She thinks about the patients she is seeing after lunch, especially the pregnant teenager, still underage. Will she manage to finish school? To take proper care of her baby and still get an education?

The general practitioner tries to suppress her feeling that Zac's worries about his heartrate variability are trivial and egocentric in comparison. She is Zac's doctor too, and she is obliged to show all her patients respect. Will Zac not feel rejected if she comes across as uninterested in his printouts? In her experience, patients who bring their self-monitoring results with them always have this look of 'this time you really MUST recognise the pattern in my data'. The general practitioner leans back in her chair, seeking a position that eases the dull pain in her head, before she starts to read, still uncertain about what she can do to help Zac.

Interpretation and health

According to commonly promoted ideals, in the narrative above Zac is behaving as a responsible citizen. By exercising every day and by seeking expert help to interpret the signals from his body when in doubt, he takes his health seriously. Zac has collected information about his body through a regime of technical devices (e.g. pulse monitoring) and structured accounts of his sensations (e.g. headache diary). He then seeks help from medical expertise to judge the meaning of these data and to receive advice about how to respond to his symptoms. One can see that Zac's management of his health aligns strongly with the cosmology of surveillance: the more information, the better. The ultimate form of surveillance is self-surveillance. This also means that we can regard Zac as a demonstration of the fully medicalised and quantified self (Vogt et al., 2016). In what might be termed the cosmology of self-surveillance, the self is the product and producer of continuous measurements that must refer to an external authority for interpretation. However, while Zac in one sense is behaving like a responsible citizen, taking public health recommendations very seriously, there is also something unnerving and even heart-rending about his predicament. It is unnerving because Zac can never rest. There is always a possibility that his body is failing him. It cannot be trusted. Zac must always monitor his own body, and he cannot even be sure that his current repertoire of self-surveillance includes the exact data that is needed in order to discover problems early enough. This is distressing and heart-rending because we get a sense that the lack of spontaneity and trust in Zac's relationship with himself is somehow unhealthy. Knowing that, although consistently and with great effort striving for what appears to be a noble goal, Zac may actually be heading for the exact opposite of what he wishes to achieve, his attitude and behaviour verges on the tragic.

Doctors, by professional training, tend to look for problems, symptoms, and to think of symptoms as the ways in which pathological processes within the human organism rise to the surface so that patients become aware of these processes and can seek help. The doctor's task, on seeing the patient and learning about his symptoms, is to identify and (hopefully) to correct the faulty process, remove the pathology. This seems to be what the French surgeon René Leriche is referring to in his dictum written in 1936, stating that '[h]ealth is life lived in the silence of the organs' (Canguilhem, 1989, p. 91; 2008). In other words, as long as the organs keep silent, we are healthy. Once the organs are no longer silent, once they whisper or cry out that something is wrong, we go to the doctor and expect him to diagnose what is wrong and to fix it.

Experience, however, teaches us all that reality is not quite that simple. Our organs are never truly silent. We permanently live with-in-through myriads of sensations that arise in-from-through the body. So how, then, can people recognise the difference between a symptom of pathology and a non-pathological sensation? This is an aspect of the question of how to distinguish pathology from normality, the elusive question that occupied the French philosopher of science George Canguilhem.

Canguilhem took up and problematized Leriche's claim that health is the state of affairs 'in the silence of the organs'. According to Canguilhem, we need a norm in order to distinguish the normal from the pathological (Canguilhem, 1989). Canguilhem hypothesises that all living beings have the capacity to interpret their inner status and its relationship with their surroundings and to make adjustments to maintain their own health (Canguilhem *et al.*, 2012). On this account, the question becomes; when is my situation of such a nature that I need external help to maintain my health? When are my own capacities for adjustment surpassed? With current high levels of medicalisation, it seems that people's intuitive ability to interpret and adapt their own embodied situation is no longer trusted, neither by health authorities, nor by the medical community, practitioners or the individual herself.

As our demands for good health increase, and with the rise of risk/surveillance medicine, listening for symptoms becomes more demanding and frustrating. Since we now have technical methods to increase our ability to record what has previously been inaudible, such as the activity of our organs, often providing us with quantitative information about them, the implication seems to be that every bodily sensation potentially is a sign of malfunction, and that our spontaneous (interpretative) self-experience is not to be trusted. On this view, there is always reason to be suspicious of one's body. One should listen attentively and with suspicion, always expecting (potential) pathology to make itself heard.

Seen from philosopher Michael Foucault's angle, the consequence of a situation where the individual person is encouraged to see herself more from the outside, with a clinical gaze, as it were, as much as or more than as a self-understanding self in the Taylorian sense of the term is that the way a human being turns him- or herself into a subject is changed:

> Having internalized the discourse of medicine existent in the community at large, the subject is able to engage in self-diagnosis and self-identification … the subject must be in a constant state of guardedness regarding the possible encroachment of disease. Further, the subject must possess an ability to determine the presence of disease, but the subject, like the physician, cannot be sure of an exact interpretation of felt body abnormalities.
>
> (Spitzack, 1992, p. 55)

In our experience, general practitioners frequently meet people like Zac who consult out of fear that a minor sensation can be a symptom of imminent illness.

We see that people feel alienated and distrusting of their bodies due to sensations that they could probably have ignored or somehow accepted or adapted to without medical intervention. It seems that people increasingly lack the confidence to spontaneously interpret and adapt to their sensations.

A further problem can then arise in this situation if, as frequently occurs, the general practitioner is stranded at the biomedical pole, to borrow an expression from Iona Heath (1999). In the current professional and societal climate, the pressure on the general practitioner not to miss any disease is strong. Fear of disease and fear of false negatives drives extensive investigations (Heath, 2014). Of course, this sometimes leads to positive findings, be they true or false. The main catch is, however, that the doctors' biomedically oriented search for disease can easily intensify the patients' distrust of their bodies and engender dysfunctional responses, not least when their symptoms are not related to specific illnesses amenable to biomedical management in the first place. Distrust and thus disjunction between mind (as source or locus of interpretation) and body (as source of experience and locus of response) may consequently escalate.

Based on the above we first suggest that virtually any aspect of our embodied existence can give rise to serious illness and suffering. Any pain in the neck or shoulder, if we persistently interpret it as a dangerous or threatening symptom and respond by contracting antagonistic muscles in the chest and neck, can become chronic, adding layer upon layer of non-adaptive interpretations and responses, intensifying and solidifying until non-reversible and perhaps even all-consuming. Any sensation of bloating and abdominal cramps, compounded over time by sufficient layers of enduring fight-or-flight responses, and by interpretations involving fear, low self-esteem or embarrassment, can become an incapacitating condition. Any sensation, if not interpreted and adapted to in a sufficiently functional manner, can become a source of non-helpful fear, retraction, social isolation, embarrassment or disintegration. It seems probable that the cosmology of self-surveillance increases the likelihood of people falling into such vicious circles.

Our second suggestion is that there is always the danger that the doctor's response to the story told and the signs revealed will diminish the patient's ability to manage her own embodied existence. If the doctor performs excessive investigations of minor symptoms, or encourages the patient to return immediately if new symptoms arise, this may confirm to the patient that there is ample reason to suspect something serious is the matter with her, and that she has insufficient resources to take care of her own health. A second MRI of the shoulder of the patient in the example in the paragraph above, further blood tests, dietary instructions, or advice to reduce his alcohol consumption – these are all examples of instances where the general practitioner takes on the role of the one who knows what is best for the patient in non-acute medical situations, while the patient's role is that of the recipient of favours he would have been unable to grant himself. In addition to the above mentioned danger of increased worries, there may be elements of dependency and disempowerment in such a relationship, even in cases where the parties agree that the patient's renewed strength and good health is what they both aim at. If unbalanced, the biomedical model increases the likelihood of general practitioners contributing to such vicious circles.

How, then, may these less than beneficial tendencies be countered? Perhaps, if we are fully to accept that our existence is one of embodied selves, as Merleau-Ponty has suggested, we need to acknowledge that embodiment entails an enduring task of interpretation, incessantly sorting out what our body tells us. Life involves an endless flux of sensations, all of which we may potentially interpret as either signs of the temporary success of life or symptoms of pathology. Through and through, our experience of our own existence comes through bodily sensations. Furthermore, when assigning meaning to what is going on with ourselves, in us and in our surroundings, we continuously have to perform this interpretation in light of moral values: Is this good or bad? Desirable or not? How to react? How to engage with our surroundings? All of these questions eventually have a moral side to them. We cannot judge the meaning of anything that affects us except by relating it to the values that organise our thoughts and actions (Laitinen, 2002; Ricoeur, 2013; Taylor, 1989). So the question of whether something is a symptom of disease or not, whether the general practitioner should initiate a search for disease or not, cannot be resolved without reference to fundamental moral values. Health is a moral state of affairs, says Gadamer (1996, p. 20).

We can now describe Zac's situation as involving a problem of interpretation, where Zac himself does not feel confident that he has access to the value codes needed to perform the interpretation of his sensations. In fact, it is rather unlikely that Zac relates his symptoms as such to values at all. As if they were troubling him without really being of him, Zac himself seems to have no way of determining whether the sensations coming from his body are a sign of illness or not. Zac does not comprehend what is going on with himself. Instead, he detaches the symptom from himself as a person, and plots them, surveillance style, into his forms and calendars. Bringing his self-surveillance results to his general practitioner, Zac has deferred the authority to judge the meaning of his own embodied experience to an external authority.

A further feature of the case of Zac is that the information that Zac asks his general practitioner to interpret consists of quantified measurements and factual accounts only. The result of Zac's self-surveillance is impersonal. It is not a story with a moral agent in it. Rather, it is a story with nobody in it, and the request is consequently that she interprets a story about nobody. This may be part of the reason why the general practitioner feels disheartened by Zac's request that she read his report.

If Zac's general practitioner is stranded at the biomedical pole, it is unlikely that she can offer him a satisfactory answer. For, as all her tests prove, nothing indicates that Zac is ill in a way that would helpfully be conceptualised and managed in biomedical terms. On the other hand, if her perspective is broader than the strictly biomedical one, she may come to ask herself and Zac different questions about his troubles.

The physician and philosopher Eric Cassell writes, 'Because humans are of a piece and *whatever happens to or is done to one part affects the whole*, sickness inevitably involves the entire person, every single part' (Cassell, 2013). If this is the case, Zac's shoulder with its painful sensation and his head with its headache must be seen as aspects of Zac and who he is in an existential sense. To merely regard them as (mechanical) body parts, would then be a violation and an alienation of Zac as a whole, as a self. Yet, this is very much how responsible citizens in late modernity have learnt to regard themselves; public campaigns about life style, health, and self-surveillance are to a high degree directed towards maintenance of the body, whilst detached from ourselves as selves. The body we are encouraged to maintain is presented as a separate unit, as something other than the self.

Zac does his best to be a responsible citizen, as most people do. He is well aware of public health advice about e.g. physical activity, wholesome food, and temperance with regard to alcohol. In addition to giving him pleasure, then, Zac's training may be regarded a sign that he is attempting to do what is right and good. In fact, by devoting so much of his attention to training, Zac has chosen one of the most powerful ways of showing this in a society and a time where fitness and self-surveillance are promoted as something every citizen should aim at, and where such capacities thus are closely connected to morality. Indeed, the emphasis on these capacities is such that by cultivating them one gets close to what would in earlier days be termed virtues; temperance, endurance, responsibility. Consequently, when Zac feels pain and has to reduce his training scheme, he is less capable of doing what he feels is right and what he therefore ought to do. As a person used to regarding himself as conscientious and responsible, where does this leave Zac if he cannot display these capacities in the way he has usually displayed them?

When Taylor claims the need for meaning to be inherent to us as persons, he adds that meaning is established on the grounds of values. What we value is linked to our sense of who we are, then, and our values are fundamentally dependent on our surroundings; on the dominating ideas in our time and our culture, as well as on other people's views and direct response to us (Taylor, 1985). If we relate this to the above statements about promoting health through (self-)surveillance, physical exercise, diet, etc., we may be getting a fairly accurate view of core values in Western late modernity, at least as seen by a secular, educated middle-class citizen like Zac. Understood thus, it is not strange that Zac is worried it has become more difficult to keep his training scheme up. It is also not strange that he wants his general practitioner to find an explanation of his pain – preferably one that comes with a solution. Who would he be, if he has to reduce his exercise programme?

We have argued that we are nothing if not our body, that the self is embodied. Yet, although we are entirely dependent on it, we are more than the sum of our organs. In coherence with Taylor's claim that we as selves are self-interpreting, meaning-seeking beings, it is our conviction that we cannot build a framework of values solely on our biological, bodily existence. We need a broader understanding of ourselves and a broader range of values on which we can establish a meaningful life; otherwise, we will be ill served as persons.

In Taylor's view 'there is a direct connection between what one values and who one is; and what one values depends on one's beliefs about what human beings are or should be' (Maicher, 2008, p. 53). Maybe this is where it goes wrong for Zac. Maybe he has internalised contemporary ideas about exercise and self-surveillance as a major part of what gives his life a direction and meaning, without even thinking too much about it.

Could it be more helpful for Zac to reflect on why his pain worries him so much, rather than to doggedly continue the search for a biomedical explanation? A general practitioner not stranded at the biomedical pole, but aware of the patient as a person, might want to take a broad view on Zac's worries. Rather than continue along the track that has proved unfruitful, she might ask him (in a manner as concrete as possible) what his values are. What is important to him? What is he hoping to achieve? Where does he belong? What are the circumstances, who are the actors and what are the values that inhabit his life-world, and how does he see his own endeavours within this context?

To be sure, it may be satisfactory to exercise, and it is not difficult to understand that Zac values this. Yet, would Zac agree that fitness is his moral basis, if confronted with a suggestion that he acts as though this is the case? That seems unlikely. It seems far more likely that, given the chance to discuss it, Zac would list a number of other values. For example, his family is very dear to him. He might also mention the fact that it is important to him to act and reason as a responsible individual and citizen. Being unable for the moment to pursue the discussion with Zac, it seems right to withhold any further suggestions about how Zac might combine his sports interest with his roles as a father and as a responsible citizen. Maybe he wants to volunteer as a coach on his kids' football team? Or something totally different.

The point is that Zac might come to see that some values are more important to him than others are, as might most of us if challenged on the topic of our values. If so, perhaps Zac can come to see his muscular pain as bearable. Standing on a moral ground that is somewhat more firm, he could find in himself a confidence that there is nothing serious the matter. After reminding himself of his basic stand that there are other things to life than training, he might find it possible to endure a pain that certainly disturbs him, but which may at the same time be seen simply as a reminder that he has been exercising and treating his body to the very limits of what it can endure.

Case two: Fred who is unemployed and a single parent

Fred is 49 years' old. He is the single father of two teenagers, and he has been unemployed for four years. Fred and his girls live in an urban area where most people's educational and income levels are low. Fred likes beer and American cars. Although the only car he can afford nowadays is a small Fiat, Fred dreams of a Buick. 'Some day...!' Fred tells himself. When Fred was a toddler, his father worked in heavy industry, but he lost his job when Fred was about ten years old. In the years after he lost his job, Fred's father increasingly took to the bottle. Because of the memories of this, Fred himself tries to be vigilant about drinking.

Recently, Fred has felt disturbed and humiliated by the procedures he must go through at the Job Centre to prove that he is eligible for Jobseekers Allowance. The people there remind him of how he felt as a teenager when he got the impression from some of his teachers that he was a nuisance and that he himself was to blame for his failures. When Fred complained that his desperate situation was 'driving him to the edge', a friend of his suggested that it was about time to visit a doctor.

When he consults with his general practitioner whom he has not met before, Fred complains that he has been feeling 'drained'. It's hard to see why, Fred comments. For although there are the girls to take care of, it's still not as though he exhausts himself. It's not that hard to keep the flat in order, and the daily shopping round is also easy work. As for jobs, well, Fred finds there really aren't many around to even apply for.

The doctor asks Fred to fill out a PHQ-9 to find out if he is depressed, commences to measure his blood pressure, and orders blood tests. At a subsequent appointment, Fred learns that the results from the questionnaire indicate that he may be depressed, and that the HbA1C measurement shows that he has developed pre-diabetes.

A couple of months later, sitting in the waiting room before another appointment for his pre-diabetes, Fred senses a humiliation about seeing his GP similar to the one he has felt at the Job Centre.

At the same time, the general practitioner readies herself before calling Fred in. She casts a glance at Fred's most recent lab results on the computer screen. She notices that Fred's HbA1C and weight have not improved. She takes a deep breath and makes a mental note to inform Fred that she is going to refer him for an exercise and weight loss programme. The general practitioner's past performance in treating patients with type two diabetes is excellent, and she is definitely not going to do an inferior job at dealing with pre-diabetes. With determination the doctor gets on her feet, walks to the door and opens it. In the waiting room Fred is reading a paper. 'Good morning,' the doctor says cheerfully. 'Please come in!'

Being at risk

When the general practitioner responds to Fred's distress and exhaustion, in addition to suggesting blood tests, she asks Fred to fill out the PHQ9 and subsequently informs him that he suffers from a mild depression. Initially, it was Fred's feeling drained that made him decide to see his general practitioner. However, in the ensuing discussion about the PHQ-9 score and about how to respond to Fred's depression, his experience of enduring distress, humiliation and powerlessness are not part of the topic, and neither are the specific circumstances of Fred and his family – the very circumstances that Fred is trying to cope with. Is it at all possible for the general practitioner to offer Fred adequate help when she ignores this? We think not, and we will elaborate this position below. Before that, we take a closer look at the course the general practitioner chooses to mark out for Fred.

The diagnosis 'pre-diabetes' is a recent invention, as is the strongly over-lapping condition 'impaired glucose tolerance'. The significance of pre-diabetes and impaired glucose tolerance is that some people described by these diagnoses develop type 2 diabetes. However, neither pre-diabetes nor impaired glucose tolerance carry any symptoms. They are asymptomatic 'risk conditions', different from the ailments that previously used to bring people to their general practitioner. Actually, they are what one might call second-order risk conditions because mild diabetes type 2 usually does not carry any symptoms either. People with mild diabetes are at a somewhat higher risk of developing symptoms, and a proportion of those who develop symptoms go on to develop serious complications, but those at the mild end of diabetes type 2 still do not have any symptoms.

Therefore, what Fred has, is a risk of developing a risk of developing a disease. A strange diagnosis indeed, and a dubious one, because the benefits of screening and treatment are far from certain, while the costs are high and the amount of harm considerable (Simmons *et al.*, 2012; Yudin and Montori, 2014).

Today, people who are in good health are urged to visit general practices and pharmacies to find out whether they have diabetes or are 'at risk'. Those who receive a diagnosis are encouraged to follow lifestyle advice and to visit general practice at regular intervals for follow-up. On top of this, those with diabetes usually receive drugs. The diagnosis of diabetes and its precursor conditions depends on laboratory measurements only, and the success or failure of treatment is defined in terms of regular laboratory measurements. Thus, the epidemic of type 2 diabetes and its precursor conditions is based on the biomedical cosmology of surveillance and laboratory measurements. And, clearly, since the diagnosis, surveillance and treatment of each of these conditions is based on measurements and judgements made by the doctor without reference to the subjective experience of the patient, the management of type 2 diabetes and its precursor conditions is also object-oriented.

Let us now return to Fred who has been informed by his general practitioner that he has pre-diabetes. What does this information mean to Fred? Is the diagnosis useful? Will it, for example, in any way help him to feel less drained? We do not know, but we fear that the diagnosis may not be particularly helpful to Fred, and that it may even have a contrary effect. To do something about a risk condition without symptoms, Fred is advised to change his life style. Eat differently, begin to exercise, lose weight. Quite a task. It is not at all certain that Fred will manage to meet the general practitioner's demands, especially since he is at the same time left to himself with regard to his unemployment, his loneliness and his struggles as a single father. It could all easily lead to a strengthened feeling of the humiliation Fred remembers from school, and which he now feels when he comes to the Job Centre or his general practitioner. Fred's self-interpretation, his understanding of himself as a fellow who does not cope particularly well or quite simply as a failure may easily be confirmed or even strengthened. Thereby, the GP's focus on what she regards measurable and quantifiable entities may be unhelpful or downright harmful. Thereby, Fred may well be at risk, but it is not at all certain that the major threat is the one his GP is focusing on.

The epidemiology of disadvantage

Any GP should know that social inequality goes hand in hand with poorer health. Yet, it seems as though Fred's doctor does not find this relevant to the way she should treat Fred. The fact is that deprivation is a strong predictor of health problems. We know from epidemiological studies that people like Fred are at increased risk of many different diseases due to deprivation. This holds true not only for absolute deprivation from basic material goods such as shelter and food, but also for relative deprivation, and for deprivation along the dimensions of culture and sociality. Among the numerous epidemiological studies that have demonstrated that a position towards the bottom of social hierarchies is detrimental to health, the British Whitehall studies are some of the best known. There is really no better way of taking in the strong link between disadvantage and poor health than from the words of Sir Michael Marmot:

> people at the bottom of the hierarchy had a higher risk of heart attacks. Secondly, it was a social gradient. The lower you were in the hierarchy, the higher the risk. So it wasn't top versus bottom, but it was graded. And, thirdly, the social gradient applied to all the major causes of death ... to cardiovascular disease, to gastrointestinal disease, to renal disease, to stroke, to accidental and violent deaths, to cancers that were not related to smoking as well as cancers that were related to smoking – all the major causes of death.
> (Marmot, 2002)

This is a striking consequence of inequality indeed. The causal mechanisms need elucidation. Sometimes, disadvantage translates into behaviour that is clearly harmful to health. This is currently the case with smoking, which for some time has been much more common among people of lower socioeconomic status in many societies. However, the social gradient in health does not disappear in the Whitehall studies or in other studies even if known risk factors such as smoking are taken into account. More subtle mechanisms seem to be in play. One assumes that this has to do with how subjective experience affects our biology. Social status that is negatively valued is also negative for health. Marmot elaborates this point:

> Human values ... I think, are absolutely crucial here. But I'm also interested in empirical demonstration of how they translate into pathology, because in the end people go and get sick, and a value sounds like something rather abstract – that it's the mind, where, in fact, what happens in the mind has a crucial impact on what happens in the rest of the body. The mind is part of our biological makeup as well. So the empirical study is how the sets of

values translate into people's perception of reality, and that, in turn, changes physiology and leads to risk of disease. So we're trying to deal in a crude way with a mind-body question of how the one translates into the other.

(Marmot, 2002)

The glimpse we have of Fred's life suggest that he and his daughters live towards the bottom of society in more than one sense. To be sure, there must be some patches of sun in his life. We do not hear of any major concerns for the girls, for example, and we can hope that his children bring Fred more joy than worries. Still, based on what we know about the epidemiology of disadvantage, there is a strong argument that Fred is in danger of developing long-term health problems.

At first sight, this indicates that Fred's general practitioner has good reason to seek to prevent Fred from developing diabetes, and to investigate whether Fred may be depressed. Depression and diabetes alongside the different life-threatening diseases and complications associated with diabetes are among the problems that people are more likely to incur if they are disadvantaged. The general practitioner thus seems to provide help that could be of great consequence since it may prevent Fred from suffering serious illness in the future. It also looks as if by making this big effort for Fred his general practitioner also laudably attempts to reduce social gradients in health among her patients. Surely, those who are underprivileged deserve that general practitioners seek to treat or – even better – to prevent the illnesses that they are more likely to incur as underprivileged.

However, despite the doctor's (presumed) good intentions, the consultations with her make Fred feel powerless and worthless. For the general practitioner does not really respond to Fred's moral plea. She fails to address Fred's feeling that his life is at a dead end, and neither does she acknowledge the adversity of Fred's life situation, the relationship between that situation and Fred's feelings of dread and exhaustion, or the threat this situation poses for Fred's health and wellbeing. She goes as far as to offer impersonally delivered mental techniques for Fred's depression, in addition to initiating quantified surveillance for Fred's asymptomatic risk for diabetes. That is all. By so doing, the doctor treats Fred as an object. She does not take Fred seriously as a person. This is unethical, of course. In addition, the doctor's behaviour confirms Fred's view of himself as an unimportant, uninteresting person, and so harms his already fragile self.

Re-interpretation, coherence and a changed self

In Taylor's view, self-interpretation, self-understanding and self-narrative are all necessary to establish the sense of self which he regards a basic condition of being a person. This sense is significant and decisive for our way about our life-world even when the narrative is one about loss or weakness. Taylor regards self-interpretation, based on our own story about ourselves, as a means to ascribe meaning to the past and direction to the future (Abbey, 2004, pp. 38–9; Taylor, 1989, pp. 47, 50–2). The story can be contributory to the current situation, even if it is in some respects an erroneous one, and a sad story can have as much power as a 'map' for the direction we choose to follow into the future as a story about, say, success or accomplishment. This does not mean that all self-narratives are equally useful. In Fred's case, for example, there seems to be a possibility that his self-narrative is to an undue degree evolving into one about shortcoming and perhaps even failure. There is a danger of the general practitioner's confirming such a story by the way she tackles his concerns. In that case, her attitude is less than helpful for Fred.

Sometimes, we feel as though life is mostly about getting through the day. At such times, to live is to exist, little more. This is about where Fred currently finds himself. At other times, by contrast, we feel that we really lead a life that is both meaningful and gratifying. This sense of leading a life is, among other things, a matter of health and well-being, and so relates to Anton Antonovsky's salutogenic model and this model's concept 'sense of coherence', which Antonovsky defined as

> a global orientation that expresses the extent to which one has a pervasive, enduring though dynamic feeling of confidence that (1) the stimuli deriving from one's internal and external environments in the course of living are structured, predictable and explicable; (2) the resources are available to one to meet the demands posed by these stimuli; and (3) these demands are challenges, worthy of investment and engagement.
>
> (Antonovsky, 1987, p. 19)

Antonovsky thought that as far as possible doctors should promote people's sense of coherence rather than focus on illness, symptoms and (potential) risk factors. To promote the sense of coherence means to focus on capacity and meaningfulness, not on what is defect or in decline. The sense of coherence has three components; meaningfulness, comprehensibility and manageability (Antonovsky, 1996, p. 15). Meaningfulness relates to a wish and motivation to cope, that things are really worthwhile, that our day to day life is interesting and a source of satisfaction, and that there is therefore good reason or purpose to care about what happens. Comprehensibility has to do with a sense that you can understand events in your life and reasonably predict what will happen in the future, and that it is therefore possible to understand and tackle the challenges we face. Manageability is a term for the belief that we have the skills, the ability, the support, the help, or the resources necessary to take care of things, and that things are manageable and within your control. Christopher Dowrick returns to these themes in Chapter 6.

Fred is not asked about his wish or motivation to cope. His doctor does not discuss the everyday challenges in his life with him. She does little to support him in making sense of his situation and less to help him take control over things. Instead, she uses tests and forms that make little sense to Fred. The test results are incomprehensible to him without help from the doctor, who not only has little to offer with regard to the worries that brought Fred to her surgery in the first place, but who also informs him that he has problems Fred himself had no idea about. In this sense, what takes place between Fred and his general practitioner is practically the opposite of salutogenesis. It is, to borrow a term from Ricoeur, a violation, which he contrasts with morality (Ricoeur, 2013, pp. 35–40).

The moral alternative, according to Ricoeur, would have been to help Fred (re-)establish coherence, specifically by emphasising capacities rather than hindrances (Ricoeur, 2005), and thus promote his sense of 'leading a life'. Like Taylor, Ricoeur thinks articulation and narrative are vital elements in such a process. However, to Ricoeur, it also matters that we as persons become aware of our potential, what we are capable *agents*, i.e. as acting individuals (cf. Latin *agere*, which means to act), and thus place ourselves in the role of the protagonist of our own story. This, of course, means that we need to take on responsibility for our life, yet also to realise that this responsibility has its limits, as Ricoeur argues (2005, pp. 104–9). All of this is part of what it means to Ricoeur to *recognise oneself*, which seems to be something that can be helpful in a situation like Fred's. We also believe, however, that this task may sometimes seem unsurmountable, and that we may then need some support, perhaps even from professionals.

Taylor claims that our self-interpretation is constitutive for who we are, but he also makes it clear that although the self-interpretation is constructed *by* the self, it is not in all regards *of* the self. As stated above, how we see ourselves is also shaped by how we are seen by others and relate to them. This means that our understanding of ourselves is influenced by external factors, such as other people, also when we are not always conscious of it. Consequently, interaction with others and our behaviour towards each other matters a great deal, particularly when we are in a position where other people depend on us.

When the doctor dismisses the concern that matters most to Fred, she fails to treat him as a person. She thereby confirms the negative strands in his self-image, when what he needs is encouragement and a sense of coherence. Given that our identity is influenced by others and the way they relate to us, the doctor's non-response to Fred's worries is a confirmation of their – and thereby his own – unimportance. In his own way, Fred is a stayer and definitely a decent father in spite of finding himself and his family in a difficult position without the promise of any escape. Maybe what Fred needs most simply is for the doctor to bear witness to his difficulties, his endurance and his courage. However, this is not what Fred gets. Instead of some simple words of solace, the doctor's focus on tests forces him to face the image of an unemployed, depressed man with prediabetes. It is not at all certain that this is particularly helpful.

Each autobiography is not a static narrative. We develop and change our story as our life proceeds and as our circumstances change. Yet, since the community, too, is constitutive of the person and self-interpretations are drawn from interchanges on both the individual and the over-individual level (Taylor, 1989), our self-interpretation may also change if we are offered other people's interpretation of our story, always (a bit) different from our own version. It is Taylor's conviction that re-narrations and re-interpretations may be life changing. By understanding ourselves in new and different ways, we change as people (Abbey, 2004). Hence, reinterpretations of the self and revisions of the autobiographical narrative in fact entails 'changes in what man is, such that he has to be understood in different terms' (Taylor, 1985, p. 55). This is a powerful claim. If it holds true, first, much may be achieved by means of doctors' co-interpretation of their patients' narratives, provided that the doctor is a skilled listener and interpreter. Second, if narratives and interpretations are decisive for our self-understanding and our means to live a good life, they should definitely be taken seriously. What we do *not* do may then matter as much as what we do, as Fred's story demonstrates. We will return to these points in the discussion of the following case story, that of Theresa.

The claim that changes in the way we understand ourselves change who we are, resembles the hypothesis at heart of narrative medicine (e.g. Burton and Launer, 2003; Launer, 2002) which indeed has much in common with the theories of Taylor, Ricoeur and Antonovsky referred to in this section. Although neither Ricoeur nor Taylor is focusing on health in particular, but on human self-understanding in general, health is a core issue for many aspects of our lives and so of our self-understanding. Especially when we are *dis-eased*, in Antonovsky's terminology, the story about our health may tend to be a very central part of the story about ourselves and to have considerable impact on our understanding of who we are.

Case three: Theresa, a woman in persistent pain

Theresa is 39 years' old. She is divorced and currently lives in a small flat in the town where she also works. Theresa has no children. For some years now, Theresa has worked part time as a receptionist for an investment bank. Theresa is not the outgoing type. Her means are limited, so she could not afford that sort of life style anyway. Smart clothes, makeup, eating out, expensive shows or concerts – nothing of that is within reach, Theresa feels. It is fortunate, she tells herself, that she enjoys good TV shows and films. Lately, she has also taken up knitting and often knits as she watches TV. Although Theresa sometimes shares a bottle of wine or a meal with her neighbour who is single like herself, she spends most of the time in her own company.

As long as Theresa can remember, she has had some health issue or other. She has for many years suffered from pain in her throat and face and from episodes of malaise. When in her early 20s, Theresa went through extensive neurological examinations. At that time, Theresa was unable to pursue her studies due to intense pain that was accompanied by visual disturbances. The medical examinations came to nothing, and no one has been able to explain the source of the pain, nor to cure it, since then.

On top of this, Theresa suffers from eczema and chronic low-grade sinusitis. Two years ago, she went through a surgical procedure that was supposed to relieve her sinusitis. However, although CT-scans indicate that the drainage of Theresa's sinuses has improved since the surgery, her symptoms have not subsided. Nowadays, Theresa occasionally buys opioids and benzodiazepines illegally for the pain in her throat and face.

Theresa's current general practitioner is aware that Theresa has reported to previous healthcare staff that her uncle abused her sexually when she was in her teens. However, this topic has not come up in any conversation that the general practitioner has had with Theresa. Actually, the general practitioner feels a bit intimidated by Theresa. He generally finds it rather difficult to relate to patients with chronic pain. Chronic and 'unexplained' pain are among the clinical problems in general practice that he dislikes. However, when it comes to Theresa, he thinks to himself, perhaps it all comes down to her drug issue. The general practitioner is determined he is going to motivate Theresa to try an internet-based programme for drug abuse the next time she visits.

Inscribed bodies

Theresa's doctors have investigated and sought to treat her pain from the (non-existing) 'point of nowhere', assuming that the subjective experience of the person in pain is of little relevance. According to the work of the German-Norwegian general practitioner and researcher Anna Louise Kirkengen, this is a grave mistake.

Through a career spanning more than 40 years, Kirkengen has gathered evidence of how traumatic experience of sufficient severity or duration to violate personal integrity leads to serious and long-lasting adversity to health. Traumatic lifetime experiences can adversely affect health through pathways that do not respect the mind-body dualism that is inherent in the biomedical model. According to Kirkengen, biomedical management of patients who suffer long-term consequences of integrity violations fails to provide adequate help and can even perpetuate and compound the adversity. When we suffer health problems due to violations of our embodied selves, a model that ignores subjectivity and fails to link body with selfhood is a failure (Kirkengen, 2010).

Kirkengen initially collected stories that her patients in general practice confided to her. Later on, she has systematically explored such individual stories and the profound and life-long damage that violation of integrity can cause. Alongside collecting and analysing individual stories, Kirkengen has synthesised available epidemiological evidence of the adversity of violation to health. Finally, she has established from phenomenological and biomedical evidence elements of a theoretical model that explains how persons who early in life experience physical, sexual and psychological violations develop serious health problems. At the core of this model of the lived experience of violation is the assumption that the lived body in the first person singular (as well as in its plural relations) should be the object matter of medicine rather than the impersonal body in the third person (cf. Leder, 1990b; Merleau-Ponty, 1962).

According to the evidence Kirkengen has collected from epidemiology and from research at the interface between psychology, neurology and immunology, violation inscribes itself in the body through a logic that involves the subjective meaning of the adversity for the victim. It is not possible to understand the biological consequences of subjective violation from the 'point of nowhere'. Symptoms that appear as inexplicable when analysed from an impersonal biomedical perspective, gain their meaning from the point of view of stories in which one person – a subject – suffers trauma at the hands of others.

Kirkengen also makes a strong argument that socially imposed secrecy compounds the problem. Being unable to articulate your problem, even to physicians, about abuse, can intensify the violation. Taboos are by their very nature hard to break. Even if someone has abused you, which transgression clearly involves breaking a taboo, and you have a strong need to disclose this trauma to others in order to seek help, your need to tell others about the abuse will in most cases be hampered by the same taboo. However, Kirkengen states that secrecy is not the sole or even the strongest reason why seeking help can become a further violation for those suffering health consequences of abuse. The fundamental conundrum is that within the medical cosmology of objectivity, where subjective experience should be left aside in order to ascertain objective truth, there is no place for the lived experience of violation. When we methodologically eliminate people's experience and give priority to objective signs of pathology in order to understand their problems, this cannot but become a further source of violation.

Kirkengen's earliest work focused on exploring how discrete physical, sexual and psychological violence to individuals causes health problems. Subsequently, she has extended this argument, by also referencing epidemiological evidence on the harmful effects of chronic adversity in its various forms, including 'relational or structural violence, economic hardship, loss of work, alcohol- or drug-addicted spouses, sexism or racism, or long-term care of severely diseased children' (Kirkengen, 2010, p. 36). Sudden trauma or cumulative stress that overwhelms the body's capacity to adjust to changing circumstances impairs immune and metabolic function and eventually causes illness, premature ageing and early death.

We now need to return to Theresa. How does the above relate to her and to the help she receives from her general practitioner? Kirkengen's studies indicate that basic knowledge of human, embodied nature, vulnerability, the significance of being and having a self, and of the sources of this self are prerequisites for understanding symptoms that arise due to violations of integrity. This, it seems, is where Theresa's doctor falls short. Given, at the individual level, we cannot be certain of causal relations. At the epidemiological level, however, there is plenty of evidence that trauma of the kind Theresa suffered in childhood strongly increases the risk of serious disease. In the absence of evidence of other causes, we must therefore assume that Theresa's current health problems are likely to relate to her childhood adversity.

Even if we may reasonably assume that Theresa's doctor has a certain knowledge of these matters – most people have, since this is something we acquire simply by living a life as human beings – he apparently fails to see the relevance and significance of this in his dealings with Theresa. And this does not only lead to a failure in helping the patient. According to Kirkengen, systematically ignoring Theresa's subjective experience, while investigating her problems, is likely to cause further harm. As Sally Hull and George Hull argue in relation to epistemic injustice in Chapter 1, investigations and attempts at treating her pain by methods that consistently hold Theresa's own experience as irrelevant are a way of further violating Theresa and of belittling her. As Leder points out, 'disregard for the patient's experience and life-context can lead to clinical misjudgements' (Leder, 1984, p. 37). Only by means of a clinical method that relates to Theresa as an embodied agent whose temporal biography is part of her current biology can the general practitioner help her adequately.

Theresa's story is, among other things, another example of our dialogically shaped identity. If nobody acknowledges Theresa's trauma, how can Theresa herself acknowledge it, and is it then at all possible to heal her wounds? We think not. On her own, Theresa is hardly able to relate her current problems to the traumatic experiences of her childhood. She probably needs helps to see this, as most of us would. If she on the other hand were given an opportunity to narrate her story to someone willing to acknowledge that past biography shapes current biology, Theresa might be able to see connections that have previously escaped her. The narrative context itself can have healing force, for translating experience into language means to give it a name and a shape, to be able to identify and gradually to understand it. Telling, Drew Leder claims, counteracts senselessness and isolation (Leder, 1990a), and this is one of the reasons why it may have a healing effect. Senselessness as well as isolation will be part of the problem for many of those with adverse childhood experiences. One reason for this is that the harmful experiences often involve transgression of a taboo. A taboo is somehow associated with something forbidden, but may also relate to something sacred or inviolable. The reasons why a phenomenon is regarded a taboo may vary from what an outsider would regard pure superstition to protection of the weaker party in various contexts. Incest may serve as an example of the latter. While not quite taboos in the strictest sense, other adverse childhood experiences, such as growing up with alcoholic parents or having to take care of your parents are still close to taboos since they are in strong disagreement with the concept of (healthy) family life and childhood.

Studies of childhood adversity have shown that victims of adversity are more prone than others to suffer from a number of illnesses (Kirkengen, 2010). This means that these people tend to be frequent users of health care services. If they as patients at their general practitioner's surgery or in hospital once more are treated as objects rather than as individuals who should be respected in their own right, or if their stories are rejected because of taboo, their doctors serve as agents for further violation of integrity.

Among other things by consequence of the confusing contradictions inherent to tabooed violence, Theresa does not have any strong sense of meaning nor is she able to tell a consistent story about her own life. The truth is that Theresa thinks there really is not much to tell. Not much she would want to tell, anyway. Theresa has felt ashamed of herself all her life, not just because of certain memories she has tried hard to forget, but most of all because she is such a nobody. Unnoticeable and dull. She has a part time job, to be sure, and she definitely needs the money she earns, but Theresa does not find her work fulfilling. Other people have interesting jobs, Theresa finds, whereas she has not.

Theresa's social network is limited. She has no family of her own, although she often wishes she had, and she has no close friends apart from the neighbour with whom she sometimes spends the evening. It seems fair to say that among the losses Theresa suffers we may list what Taylor has termed the affirmation of ordinary life, i.e. work and family life (Taylor, 1989), which he claims to be regarded a significant part of an individual's identity in the Western world, and so part of what makes life worth living.

One cannot expect a coherent or fully understood story from Theresa. Her entire framework threatens to collapse as a result of the conflicts and contradictions inherent to her story, the subsequent strain following her succession of illnesses, and her non-addressed impairment. Following Taylor, an unreliable framework is a threat to our identity. Without a reasonably steady framework, it is hard to know who one is. Anybody in this situation would need a reinforcement of their framework, which requires a story about one self that is at the same time a story about one's self.

Ultimately, being a self is an individual undertaking. Theresa, like the rest of us, needs to find her own way of leading a meaningful life, to recognise it as a true or faithful expression of who she is, and to adopt and take responsibility for it. However, doing a thing on one's own does not mean to do it single-handedly. That would indeed hardly be possible if selves are constructed through dialogue, as Taylor maintains. This is a given that may serve as an asset in Theresa's case since it implies that it should be possible for her doctor to take the role as co-narrator and co-interpreter. In dialogic collaboration, Theresa and her general practitioner might be able to bit by bit to construct a whole picture, the portrait of a self that by definition is a unique individual, as valuable and worthy of respect as anyone else. This might strengthen Theresa's framework and thus her capacity to lead a life, yet it is a point to which no doctor could lead her on his own. It would take Theresa's contribution all along the way to get there. Although her story is in pieces, no co-interpretation can take place unless her conversation partner knows how Theresa herself sees these pieces.

The translation into language would be a reflection of what Theresa finds inside herself, and so, the act of articulation is an act of interpretation. By narrating, Theresa would at the same time be shaping her self, her identity. The interplay between the listener's expressed reactions to what Theresa relates and her own response to these reactions may lead to new understanding that is in turn bound to change her self, according to Taylor who holds that 'any change in self-understanding will be incorporated by the individual into some sort of narrative structure about the shape and direction of his life' (Abbey, 2014, p. 276).

Before leaving Theresa, we should emphasise that it is by no means certain that a change in Theresa's understanding of herself would suffice to solve her medical problems. First, one should never take for granted that medical help can cure or fully relieve the patient's problems. Second, and even more importantly in our context, it is quite possible that Theresa will still need medications or other biomedical interventions. It is in any case essential that the general practitioner examine Theresa's problems and seek to help her both from the aspect of biography and biology. Theresa's problems are inscribed in her embodied existence. Seeking to understand and help Theresa, her doctor must move between the physiological and existential dimensions of her illness, 'understanding them as equally significant and mutually implicatory' (Leder, 2013). Getting stuck at the biographical pole would be no less inadequate than one-sidedly paying biomedical attention to the patient's problem.

Above, the main focus has been on Theresa's self-interpretation, although we have also emphasised the general practitioner's role as co-interpreter. However, the concept of interpretation is a multi-layered one in general practice. We agree with Leder who claims that medical practice is interpretative by nature and that it is imperative that doctors have interpretative skills in order to put medical science to its best use (Leder, 1990b). General practitioners use their judgment, their interpretative skills also when taking notes, when performing a physical examination of a patient, and when using diagnostic technologies (Leder, 1990a). Developing a more fully fledged account of the embodied self as the 'cosmological' principle that might underpin the interpretive nature of clinical work (Reeve, 2010) thus seems to hold great potential for general practice.

Conclusion

The patients Zac, Fred and Theresa, whose stories we have related in this chapter, all suffer. Zac's ability to make sound judgements about his own health is reduced, and he relies on professional expertise to determine how he should lead his life. Fred finds himself in a difficult situation as he has been without a job for a long time, and it takes all he has got to take care of himself and his daughters. Theresa experiences chronic pain and episodes of malaise, and the unsuccessful attempts to investigate and treat her problems, have ignored the trauma she experienced as a child. Although the three patients' life situations as well as their health problems differ, the consequences are similar for them all; their capacity to act as autonomous agents is impaired. All three present to their physicians with symptoms that are common in general practice today, and all three receive inadequate help if their problems are managed in biomedical terms only.

The object-oriented cosmology and the cosmology of surveillance are inadequate for general practice. We suggest that a theory of persons as embodied selves can serve as a better a foundation for general practice.

Key learning points

1   Patients are always more than the sum of their parts.
2   General practitioners need to constantly alternate between complementary perspectives relating to physiological and existential dimensions of illness.
3   Combining physiological and existential perspectives is hardly possible unless we adopt a medical cosmology in which we see patients as embodied subjects.

4   Seeing patients as embodied subjects enables general practitioners to better understand complex problems including the risk epidemic, the effects of social disadvantage and adverse childhood experiences on health, and 'unexplained' symptoms.

5   Concepts drawn from philosophical anthropology, in this context represented by Charles Taylor and Maurice Merleau-Ponty, can help us to achieve this.

6   Medical practice is at heart an interpretative enterprise.

References

Abbey, R. 2004. *Charles Taylor*. Cambridge, UK: Cambridge University Press.

Abbey, R. 2014. Charles Taylor: Sources of the Self. In J. Shand (ed.), *Central Works of Philosophy: Twentieth Century: Quine and After* (Vol. 5). Chesham: Acumen.

Antonovsky, A. 1987. *Unraveling the mystery of health: how people manage stress and stay well*. Jossey-Bass.

Antonovsky, A. 1996. The salutogenic model as a theory to guide health promotion. *Health promotion international*, 11 (1): 11–18.

Armstrong, D. 1995. The rise of surveillance medicine. *Sociology of Health & Illness*, 17 (3), 393–404.

Baynes, K. 2010. *Self, Narrative and Self-Construction; Revisiting Taylor's 'Self-Interpreting Animals'*. Paper presented at The Philosophical Forum.

Bentham, J. 1995. The panopticon writings. In M.B. (ed.). London: Verso.

Burton, J., and Launer, J. 2003. *Supervision and support in primary care*. Radcliffe Publishing.

Canguilhem, G. 1989. *The normal and the pathological*. New York: Zone Books.

Canguilhem, G. 2008. Health: Crude concept and philosophical question. *Public Culture*, 20 (3): 467–477.

Canguilhem, G., Geroulanos, S., and Meyers, T. 2012. *Writings on Medicine*. Bronx: Fordham University Press.

Cassell, E.J. 2013. *The nature of healing: the modern practice of medicine*. Oxford: Oxford University Press.

Engel, G.L. 1977. The need for a new medical model: A challenge for biomedicine. *Science*, 196 (4286): 129–36.

Fossland, J., and Grimen, H. 2001. *Selvforståelse og frihet: en introduksjon til Charles Taylors filosofi*. Oslo: Universitetsforlaget.

Foucault, M. 1997. *Discipline and punishment*. London: Tavistock.

Gadamer, H.-G. 1996. *The enigma of health: the art of healing in a scientific age*. Stanford University Press.

Heath, I. 1999. 'Uncertain clarity': contradiction, meaning, and hope. *British Journal of General Practice*, 49: 651–7.

Heath, I. 2011. Divided we fail. *Clinical medicine*, 11(6), 576–86.

Heath, I. 2014. Role of fear in overdiagnosis and overtreatment – an essay by Iona Heath. *BMJ*, 349. doi: 10.1136/bmj.g6123.

Jewson, N.D. 1976. The disappearance of the sick-man from medical cosmology, 1770–1870. *Sociology*, 10 (2): 225–44.

Kirkengen, A.L. 2010. *The lived experience of violation. How abused children become unhealthy adults*. Zeta Books.

Laitinen, A. 2002. Strong evaluations and personal identity.

Launer, J. 2002. *Narrative-based primary care: a practical guide*: Radcliffe Publishing.

Lea, K. 2015. *Intellectual Practicians: An Exploration of Professionalism among Upper Secondary School Teachers with Icelandic Mother Tongue Teachers as a Contextualized Empirical Case.* University of Bergen, Bergen.

Leder, D. 1984. Medicine and paradigms of embodiment. *Journal of Medicine and Philosophy*, 9 (1): 29–44.

Leder, D. 1990a. Clinical interpretation: the hermeneutics of medicine. *Theoretical Medicine*, 11 (1): 9–24.

Leder, D. 1990b. Flesh and blood: A proposed supplement to Merleau-Ponty. *Human Studies,* 13 (3): 209–19.

Leder, D. 2013. *The body in medical thought and practice* (Vol. 43): Springer Science & Business Media.

Maicher, S.G.B. 2008. *Practising culture: The concept of a practice and the critique of reductionist conceptions of culture.* PhD thesis, University of Ottawa. Available at: http://hdl.handle.net/10393/29739

Marmot, S.M. 2002) *Conversation with Sir Michael Marmot; The Whitehall Studies/ Interviewer: H. Kreisler.* Conversations with History, Institute of International Studies, University of California, Berkeley.

McWhinney, I., and Freeman, T. 2009. *Textbook of family medicine* (3rd ed.). New York: Oxford University Press.

Merleau-Ponty, M. 1962. *Phenomenology of perception.* London and New York: Routledge.

Reeve, J. 2010. Interpretive Medicine: Supporting generalism in a changing primary care world. *Occasional paper, Royal College of General Practitioners,* 88: 1–20.

Ricoeur, P. 2005. *The course of recognition* [*Parcours de la reconnaissance*] (D. Pellauer, trans.). Harvard: Harvard University Press.

Ricoeur, P. 2013. *Hermeneutics: writings and lectures, Volume 2* (D. Pellauer, trans.). Cambridge: Polity Press.

Simmons, R.K., Echouffo-Tcheugui, J.B., Sharp, S.J., Sargeant, L.A., Williams, K.M., Prevost, A.T., … and Griffin, S.J. 2012. Screening for type 2 diabetes and population mortality over 10 years (ADDITION-Cambridge): a cluster-randomised controlled trial. *The Lancet, 380* (9855): 1741–8. doi: http://dx.doi.org/10.1016/S0140-6736(12)61422-6

Smith, N.H. 2004. Taylor and the Hermeneutic Tradition. In R. Abbey (ed.), *Charles Taylor* (pp. xi, 220 s.). Cambridge: Cambridge University Press.

Spitzack, C. 1992. Foucault's political body in medical praxis. In D. Leder (ed.), *The body in medical thought and practice* (pp. 51–68). New York: Springer.

Stewart, M., Brown, J., Weston, W., McWhinney, I., McWilliam, C., and Freeman, T. 2013. *Patient-centred medicine: transforming the clinical method.* London: Radcliffe.

Taylor, C. 1985. *Human agency and language* (Vol. 1). Cambridge: Cambridge University Press.

Taylor, C. 1989. *Sources of the self: the making of the modern identity.* Cambridge: Cambridge University Press.

Taylor, C. 1992. *The ethics of authenticity.* Harvard University Press.

Taylor, C. 1995. The dialogical self. *Rethinking knowledge: Reflections across the disciplines,* 57–66.

Vogt, H., Hofmann, B., and Getz, L. 2016. The new holism: P4 systems medicine and the medicalization of health and life itself. *Med Health Care and Philos*, 19: 307–23.

Yudin, J.S., and Montori, V.M. 2014. The epidemic of pre-diabetes: the medicine and the politics. *BMJ.* doi: 10.1136/bmj.g4485.

3 Challenges to the 'self' in IT-mediated health care

Deborah Swinglehurst

Introduction

> Edith Brown (whom we have already met in the first chapter) is a 71-year-old widow who lives alone. She has numerous ongoing medical problems (atrial fibrillation, hypertension, CKD3, osteoarthritis of her right hip, recurrent depression, falls, constipation) and a history of three previous transient ischaemic attacks. She has a long list of prescribed medications (warfarin, ramipril, simvastatin, atenolol, amlodipine, paracetamol, codeine, citalopram, senna, macrogol).

Electronic patient records (EPRs) are now in widespread use in UK general practice. They present a range of opportunities to improve patient care. For example, in the care of Edith, the EPR offers facilities for quickly estimating her risk of future stroke (based on population risk tools), charting her blood pressure, prompting regular 'medication review', offering safety alerts (e.g. warning of the potential for an adverse drug interaction between simvastatin and amlodipine) and ensuring she is re-called for regular check-ups. Used wisely these functions may support her ongoing personal medical care.

EPRs and similar technologies are often presented by policymakers as the solution to many of the most complex problems in health systems such as the NHS. A recent example is the promise of significant government investment (£45 million) to support the adoption of online consultation systems (NHS England, 2016). The assumption (which is not yet supported by convincing evidence) is that these will improve patient access and efficiency in a context of rising GP workload and diminishing resources to deliver care (Casey *et al.*, 2017). Critics of this tendency towards technological determinism refer to the 'technology dream' (Oesterlund, 2002) or the 'vision of a technological utopia' (Greenhalgh *et al.*, 2009) – an imagined future in which it is mistakenly assumed that all the relevant information about a patient will be retrieved at the push of a button, making healthcare better, safer, cheaper and more integrated (Greenhalgh *et al.*, 2009). It is common for technology implementation projects to gain considerable momentum (and huge financial investment) before any attention is paid to how the technologies concerned transform roles, relationships, the distribution of work and the experience of users – in other words how they 'work' (or not) in the real world of clinical practice.

The EPR is now a rather well established technology and may seem an unpromising place to start in an enquiry into the 'self' in primary care. What can consideration of a commonplace *technology* teach us about the complexities of the human 'self'? My main point of departure in this chapter is that the EPR profoundly changes the dynamics of the clinical consultation and shapes working arrangements and relationships in significant (and sometimes unintended) ways. I see the clinical consultation, how it unfolds in its every detail, as central to the construction of 'selfhood' in the primary care setting. My experience as both a GP and as a researcher points to the EPR as being integral to the consultation and how this 'unfolding' takes shape. Close attention to how the EPR is used *in practice* may shed important light on what constitutes the 'self' and how technologies contribute in an ongoing way to shaping what it means to be a professional and a patient in primary care. Returning to Edith, a core concern is what *wise* use of the EPR in the consultation might look like, so that the 'person' we refer to when we talk about 'personal' care is not lost to the margins – and neither is the 'person' who is providing that care.

The importance of focusing on practice: what is *actually* going on?

There has been a lot of research on computers in the consulting room. Much of this research adopts an orientation towards the computer as simple technological 'data container' or 'black box' which has *impacts* on the consultation. This is surprising, since sociological research conducted in the early 1990s shows that computer use and communicative conduct are intricately coordinated (Greatbatch, 1992; Greatbatch *et al.*, 1993, 1995). For example, Greatbatch showed that patients synchronise their talk with the doctor's use of the computer, monitoring doctors' conduct to identify upcoming boundaries in keyboard use in ways that mean they can avoid interrupting the doctor's activity. Intriguingly, this research also found that patients can anticipate these boundaries *in advance of their occurrence* (by picking up subtle cues such as the shift of a doctor's gaze from keyboard to screen). When doctors are successful in 'backgrounding' their use of the computer, patients are less constrained in their interaction (Greatbatch *et al.*, 1995). Doctors' efforts at communication are similarly disrupted by the demands of their own computers. This early research was carried out when doctors were only using computers in the consultation for prescribing. GPs now spend about 40 per cent of their time interacting with the computer (Kumarapeli and de Lusignan, 2013); it is very difficult to keep the computer in the background!

So what is actually going on now that the EPR is occupying such an important role in everyday clinical work? What is being accomplished as people interact with the EPR? In my own research on the EPR I have brought a sociotechnical lens to the study of the EPR. Under this lens, people, technologies and material artefacts are seen as participating in complex interconnected networks; the focus is on the 'EPR-in-use' in everyday contexts. What comes into view is that the EPR has brought about much more radical change to the nature of 'consultation work' than that which arises from its material presence as a mere object or 'data container'. The **R**(ecord) of EPR does not *represent* the work, but is *constitutive* of the work itself (Berg, 1998). Our focus shifts towards the consideration of how the EPR contributes to shaping the practices of the professionals who interact with it, and – in turn – how these professionals shape their use of the EPR to align with their working practices. The two are intricately connected and co-evolving.

In order to unpack these complex relationships between humans and technologies in practice I have used an approach called linguistic ethnography (Creese, 2008; Snell *et al.*, 2015). Linguistic ethnography brings together close analysis of 'language-in-use' with ethnographic observation, and considers the nature and dynamics of the linkages between persons, encounters and institutions (Rampton, 2007). It involves 'zooming in' on the moment-by-moment details of the consultation and 'zooming out' to consider the wider organisational and socio-political context as co-constructed emergent phenomena. This approach has led me to conceptualise the EPR as a collection of silent but highly consequential 'voices' which profoundly shape the interaction moment-by-moment (Swinglehurst *et al.*, 2011; Swinglehurst, 2014). Some previous researchers have referred to the consultation as 'triadic', drawing attention to the patient, clinician and computer as participating in a three-way interaction, and attributing agency to the computer as an equal partner (Scott and Purves, 1996; Pearce, 2007; Pearce *et al.*, 2008, 2009). I would suggest that the EPR is both more and less than this. It delivers not one voice, but many. What it does *not* do is any of the complex social 'interaction work' that clinician and patient do to 'keep the consultation on track'. It cannot respond to the moment-by-moment nuance of social interaction. This labour necessarily falls to the clinician who must learn to weave in the additional 'voices' of the EPR without any help from the EPR in how to 'smooth things over'.

The EPR sharpens the tension between different ways of framing the patient – the patient as a unique individual with a particular narrative to share ('here and now') and a standardised, institutional version of the patient in which the patient is 'one of a population' of similar patients ('there and then'). Managing this 'dilemma of attention', which assumes different versions of the 'self', demands 'work'. How this work unfolds contributes in an ongoing way to how the 'self' (of clinician and patient) is constructed and understood.

Caring for the record, whilst caring for the patient

Arguably, the most useful contribution of the EPR is as a 'formal' tool. For example, it categorises, measures, standardises work and facilitates audit. It supports not only the management of individual patients like Edith ('primary' use of data), but produces transportable 'coded' aggregate data on things like perform-ance, costs, and other metrics ('secondary' use of data). Although the precise meaning of coded data becomes more and more difficult to interpret as the dis-tance from its original context of production increases, a considerable amount of work is invested in 'caring for the record' across general practice organisations in order to satisfy external requirements for secondary data (Swinglehurst and Greenhalgh, 2015). The EPR's facility for supporting 'secondary' use of data creates particular challenges to the construction and performance of 'selfhood' for both patient and clinician in the clinical consultation, as different versions of the 'person' compete for attention.

Formal tools have long been the subject of debate between those who see formalisation as desirable and those who see it as undesirable because it results in an impoverished version of the complex reality it seeks to represent. This tension has been called the rationality-reality gap (Heeks *et al.*, 1999) or the 'fatal paradox' between the nature of healthcare work and its standardisation (Berg, 2004). Carl May contrasts the patient as 'minimum data set' with the patient as a bearer of heterogeneous experience and narratives of ill-health (May *et al.*, 2006). Formal tools can embrace a certain 'form' of knowledge ('knowing that') but cannot replace the 'know how' or tacit knowledge, which is central to professional practice – what Polanyi calls the 'art of skilful knowing and skilful doing' (Polanyi, 1958). In a similar vein, Schön argues that the problems of greatest human concern are often *not* amenable to the instrumental problem solving approaches which constitute the model of 'tech-nical rationality' (Schön, 1983).

Technical rationality has much to offer medicine. Attempts to standardise clinical care and clinical terminology (e.g. diagnostic criteria and thresholds) and the associated metrics (such as outcomes and targets) predate the arrival of EPRs, so it would be naïve to suggest that the EPR is in some way 'causal' of this kind of activity. But the EPR also embeds 'scientific bureaucratic medicine' (Harrison, 2002), underpinned by a logic which is not only essentially algorith-mic but which also tells the clinician what 'ought to be done' (or 'what 'should be the case'). I have called this the 'deontic' voice of the EPR (Swinglehurst, 2014) and as such it constitutes a form of bureaucratic rule or social control which bears down on the consultation. The move towards a restricted range of codes to represent complex matters (for example, Edith's CKD3, depression and falls) – is not *only* about greater standardisation but is also about promoting stricter *adherence* to standards. This poses particular challenges when certain aspects of the consultation (or of patients' lives) do not 'fit' easily into boxes, or the concerns of the patient and/or clinician do not align with the bureaucratic demands that the EPR is making 'in the moment'. The question of 'whose inter-ests am I to serve?' becomes a pertinent and pressing moral question and the cli-nician needs to find ways of negotiating this. Small, apparently mundane acts of documentation in the clinic may (especially when repeated many times across an entire health system such as the NHS) have significant consequences distant to the consultation. Marc Berg cautions against becoming entrenched in arguments which pitch the 'formal' against the 'informal' (i.e. the complexity of medical work against the EPR's 'impoverished representation of it) but instead encourages a focus on 'practices' and on how skilful human beings bridge the rationality-reality gap (Berg, 1996, 1997). In this chapter we will look at some of these 'bridging' practices to see what we can learn about the professional 'self' in an environment which is increasingly adapting to the use of formal tools like the EPR, within a wider institutional context of scientific bureaucratic medicine.

The consultation, the self and the EPR

The consultation is not simply a 'formal' occasion for naming problems and measuring biological parameters. It is also an opportunity for the patient to tell their story to an 'involved' listener (Goffman, 1966) who in turn shapes the 'telling' and is witness to a patient's suffering (Berger and Mohr, 1967; Heath, 1995). Constructing narratives in the context of an ongoing therapeutic relationship is one way in which a patient may make sense of their illness in the overall context of their lived life (Charon, 2001; Greenhalgh and Hurwitz, 1999). The clinician adopts an interpretative or hermeneutic function, working with the patient to produce more hopeful or 'flourishing' narratives (Toon, 2014). Framed in this way, the concern of the consultation is with the patient's specific, unique and particular experience and with making sense of this experience in the 'here and now', in terms which are immediately relevant to the patient and sensitive to social contexts. Repeated opportunities for this 'telling' contribute to building a therapeutic relationship over time and the possibility to unleash the 'therapeutic potential' of the consultation, supporting the patient to build a coherent sense of 'self' and 'co-producing' health to the extent that this is possible in the circumstances (Balint, 1964; Toon, 2014). By 'being there' (Julian, 1987) as an active, attentive listener, the clinician offers a trusted confidential space in which the patient may rehearse different versions of their story and negotiate ways forward.

The EPR – with its propensity to favour more distal, general, standardised institutional versions of personhood and events – presents challenges to this account of the consultation and to the opportunity it offers for the construction of 'selfhood'. Professionals must learn strategies to cope with these new tensions inherent in the contemporary consultation in ways which enable them to retain (and ideally develop) their own coherent sense of 'self' whilst also helping the patient to achieve their potential. We will pursue this further later in the chapter when we take a 'close up' view of some examples of clinician-patient interaction and consider how professionals assert, perform or re-shape their professional selves in this bureaucratised context.

The work of Goffman offers some useful concepts for understanding where the EPR fits with the 'here and now' of the interaction between clinician and patient. Bakhtin helps us deal more satisfactorily with the 'distributed' nature of the EPR and the role of the EPR in delivering voices from 'out there' into the interaction. Both support an analysis which focuses on *what is being accomplished here* and both offer useful lenses for a consideration of the 'self' and how the 'self' is particularly challenged in the IT-mediated consultation. In the next section we will temporarily leave aside the EPR and look briefly at some of these useful concepts.

Introducing Goffman and Bakhtin

In *The Presentation of Self in Everyday Life* Goffman adopts a perspective of social life as theatrical performance, in which participants engage in complex displays (performances) of impression management, carefully tailored to the particular social context at hand (Goffman, 1959). The sense of self is developed through relationship with others, and on every occasion of interaction people work hard to keep this relationship on track. I will briefly introduce some of Goffman's concepts, illustrating them by reference to a short data extract from the opening of a consultation (Figure 3.1).[1]

Engagement and involvement

Goffman defines engagement/involvement as follows:

> To be engaged in an occasioned activity means to sustain some kind of cognitive and affective engrossment in it, some mobilization of one's psychobiological resources; in short it means to be involved in it.
>
> (Goffman 1966b, p. 36)

> A demand regarding engrossment is a demand on the inner spirit of the engrossed person.
>
> (Goffman 1966b, p. 38)

Crucial is the combination of the cognitive and the affective (referring to *affect* or emotional engagement) which Goffman concedes is demanding work. In Goffman's account, the assessment of involvement relies on outward expression, or on how involvement is 'allocated', although clearly the 'engrossment' sustained by an individual is a matter of inward feeling. For Goffman, *actual* involvement is inaccessible (to participants in the interaction, and indeed to the researcher analysing such interactions) but what matters in social life is the *outward expression* (or display) of involvement (Goffman, 1966). For Goffman, the 'self' *is* the 'projected self' and how the self is projected is responsive, in a nuanced, flexible and ongoing way to how the projected self is taken up in interaction with fellow interlocutors.

When the EPR is introduced into the consultation clinicians must judge how to allocate their involvement. This is not simply about where to look.

a Footing

'Footing' refers to the way in which roles and relationships of participants can change during the course of an interaction (Roberts and Sarangi, 2005; Goffman, 1981). A change in footing implies a change in the alignment (or stance or

Time	N/P	Words spoken	Bodily conduct
0.38	D	hello Mr Z* =	D looks towards door as P enters
0.39	P	=good morning	
	D	c'mon in	D raises R hand towards P
		how are you? =	D leans forward and -> EPR
0.40	P	=did you enjoy your break	D < - > P; P walking towards seat
		(0.4)	D sits back in chair, oriented towards P, crosses legs, hands to lap
0.42	D	lovely	D nods
	P	good (0.2) you deserve it	
0.44	D	ye- well we went to [name of city] so er =	P sits down. D rotates chair and turns -> EPR
0.45	P	= sorry?	P - > D; D - > EPR
0.46	D	we went to: [name of city]	D < - > P. D props head in L hand on desk.
		(0.4)	D brings hands to keyboard and looks down to keyboard
0.47	P	↑oh	
	D	it was good	
		(0.4)	
0.49	D	now how have you been	
		(0.6)	
0.50	P	well	P - > forward; D's knees under desk, head rotated (right) -> P
		(0.8)	
		It's mixed actually	D props head in L hand. P tilts head towards D, still looking forward

Figure 3.1 Illustration of involvement/engagement, footing and face-work in action.

Note
(D=doctor; P=patient).

posture or projected self) we take up to ourselves and others present, expressed in the way that we manage the production or reception of an utterance. A change in footing involves a change in our frame for events. It does not follow grammatical structures or sentence structure; it can occur over a stretch of talk which is shorter or longer than a sentence and may involve gross changes in posture or very subtle shifts in tone (Goffman, 1981).

b Face and 'face-work'

Goffman defines 'face' as 'the positive social value a person effectively claims for himself by the line others assume he has taken during a particular contact' (Goffman, 1967, p. 5). In other words it is 'a person's immediate claims about 'who s/he is' in an interaction' (Heritage, 2001). It is the outward expression of the 'self' in the moment of its expression and is distinct – but related to – more enduring aspects of a person's identity.

When two people communicate with each other they do 'face-work'. This means that they do interactional work in order to maintain their own face (ensuring an image of self which is consistent) and they are also actively *saving the face of other participants* in the interaction. The maintenance of face is therefore an inherently social, cooperative and moral affair. Each party balances their attention to the current circumstances with an eye to the social world beyond the immediate encounter.

Participants may endure threats to their own face, if there is a sense that the 'self' is being undermined by alternative inconsistent images of the self. Participants are mutually engaged in trying to avoid threats to the face of fellow participants. The flow of an interaction is dependent on this mutual attention to face by all parties. Goffman says that:

> in trying to save the face of others, the person must choose a tack that will not lead to loss of his own; in trying to save his own face, he must consider the loss of face that his action may entail for others.
>
> (Goffman, 1967, p. 14)

We will now turn to a transcript of an interaction that took place at the opening of a consultation between a GP and patient. It illustrates the richness of (apparently rather mundane) interaction as a site of intense social activity with doctor and patient collaborating in their performance of 'self-hood' moment-by-moment.

Until 0.40 the doctor and patient exchange greetings as the patient enters. The doctor asks 'how are you?' as he orients towards the EPR, but the patient does not respond, instead asking the GP about his recent break. The doctor re-orients himself in his chair, sits back, faces the patient and places his hands on his lap and says it was 'lovely' – a move which displays engagement. He goes on at 0.44 to say where he went, again re-orienting towards the EPR as the patient sits down. The patient apparently mis-hears, and demands the doctor's attention again; the doctor responds by repeating the information (this time facing the patient) and re-engaging. The doctor then brings both hands to the computer keyboard, looks down towards it, and at 0.49 asks 'now how have you been'. Here we see an obvious change in footing. The GP has not only prepared for this by placing both hands on the computer keyboard but he marks his change of footing by prefacing his question with the word 'now'. This is an example of what Gumperz calls a 'contextualisation cue' – it signals some upcoming change in roles and relationships (Gumperz, 1982, 1992).

The emphasis on the word 'you' is another example. This effects a steer away from a focus on opening pleasantries (and social 'chat' about the doctor's holiday) to a focus on the patient, and the 'official' business at hand. The patient continues, describing his recent experience with 'well (pause) it's mixed actually' and the consultation moves forward. Notice how the patient's emphasis on 'well' followed by a relatively long pause is effective in securing the doctor's engagement again (first, he rotates his head away from the EPR towards the patient, then he props his head in his hand). A change in footing has occurred. It is common for changes in footing to combine linguistic moves (e.g. emphasis, intonation) with other features, such as changes in body posture or gaze. Erickson has referred to this clustering of contextualisation cues as 'modality redundancy' and has shown that the most significant turning points in counselling interviews involve the most obvious clustering of such cues (Erickson and Shultz, 1982).

The patient's comment about the doctor's break from general practice ('good … you de<u>serve</u> it') is an example of face-work. It implies that the doctor works hard most of the time and that this should be rewarded with some time off … even if it means that he has been unavailable for appointments. The doctor similarly responds with some face-work when he replies 'ye – well we went to [name of city]'. To agree outright with the patient that he deserved a holiday (an unqualified 'yes') might be interpreted as presumptuous and immodest, but to disagree would be to suggest that the patient's remark was misplaced. Instead, we see something in between. The doctor begins with what seems like an agreement – which he self-repairs and qualifies 'ye – well' so that it becomes a partial agreement. He then offers up some limited information about his holiday, which makes clear he is happy to engage with a modicum of 'social chat', at least in the context that the patient has opened up the topic.

Bakhtin/Vološinov[2] and the 'dialogic voice'

Bakhtin describes communication as *dialogic* in nature. This concept expresses the idea that meaning is only possible at the point at which speaker and listener (or reader and writer) connect and that all spoken utterances and written texts must be understood in terms of how these utterances and texts are responding to and anticipating other utterances or texts (Vološinov, 1973; Bakhtin, 1981a). For Bakhtin, the specific meaning of words will vary depending on this immediate social context. Meaning 'is always a meeting of (at least) two minds and consciousnesses, creating results that cannot be reduced to either one of them' (1981a, p. 44; Blommaert, 2005b).

Bakhtin concerns himself not only with specific utterances but with the whole pool of utterances available to the speaker (or writer) and emphasises the importance of both the immediate and the wider social context in the interactional exchange. He says:

> the forms of signs are conditioned above all by the social organization of the participants involved and also by the immediate conditions of their interaction.
>
> (Vološinov, 1973, p. 21)

A core concept in Bakhtin's work is the notion of 'voice' as the dialogically constituted 'speaking consciousness'. Finding one's 'voice' is central to Bakhtin's conceptualisation of identity construction. He regards the 'ideological becoming' of a human being as a process of assimilating and appropriating the words of others:

> Each word tastes of the context and contexts in which it has lived its socially charged life; all words and forms are populated by intentions … the word in language is half someone else's. It becomes 'one's own' only when the speaker populates it with his own intention, his own accent, when he appropriates the word, adapting it to his own semantic and expressive intention.
>
> (Bakhtin, 1981b, p. 293)

The fundamental question for Bakhtin is 'Who is doing the talking?' When voices are reproduced they take on a new 'evaluative accent' as the speaker expresses his own intentions. Understanding depends, in turn, on what Bakhtin calls a 'responsive understanding' – which is itself also dialogic and evaluative. This sensitivity of the meaning of words to local context and evaluative accent is what lies behind concerns people may have about being misrepresented in the media, when small sections of talk are stripped of their original context and re-presented with a new evaluative accent.

How meaning is created at the point of connection between participants is related to their appreciation of 'speech genres' or socially acceptable ways of speaking in particular situations. These are relatively stable and are learnt, just as we learn language. They are an articulation of the relationship between language and culture since language is used and interpreted according to our knowledge of genres (Maybin, 2001). For example, patients who have recently arrived in the UK and who have limited English may be unfamiliar with the genre of the doctor-patient consultation in the UK primary care context and this may lead to a range of misunderstandings over and above those that arise through lack of shared vocabulary. Similarly, imagine that I bump into my patient Edith Brown in the supermarket on a Saturday morning. We are both very familiar with the social conventions around doctor-patient consultations and also the kinds of talk that arise in ad hoc meetings in supermarkets. Although we may never have met each other outside the surgery, our conversation in the supermarket will proceed very differently even if we do end up discussing Edith's health. The meaning of the words 'How are you?' in these two contexts is likely to be understood differently by both doctor and patient, and we are likely to project different versions of our 'selves', conditioned by our surroundings. For Bakhtin, it is the understanding of context (more so than *text*) that is fundamental to understand the meaning of a word. For example, it is an inherently social phenomenon (and not a matter of semantics) which results in a word such as 'wicked' acquiring a positive meaning in some contexts.

The rest of this chapter will involve looking at some examples of data illustrating clinicians at work in their consultations with patients and EPRs. Using these examples, and importing some of the social theory that we have now covered, we will consider what we can learn about the construction of 'selfhood' in the contemporary consultation. We will start with a brief look at the use of computer templates in chronic disease management (for a more detailed account see Swinglehurst *et al.*, 2012).

Nurse-led chronic disease management

The management of patients with chronic disease in UK general practice is often nurse-led and typically involves a comprehensive review of the patient undertaken on a regular basis (e.g. annually). Computer templates (highly structured electronic forms) are used to organise this work. They act as a useful aide-memoire, and as a way of establishing and documenting routines and rationalising care. They are a formal tool *par excellence*. As such they illustrate very well some of the challenges to the 'self' in the IT-mediated consultation and the strategies that clinicians use to overcome them. Many of the data items gathered in chronic disease management reviews are driven by external demands, such as the Quality and Outcomes Framework (QOF) and this is very important political context for understanding what is being accomplished in a chronic disease review.

QOF is a pay-for-performance system introduced in 2004 as part of a new national contract for general practice. It offers financial incentives to general practices for documenting a range of clinical and organisational indicators. QOF was introduced alongside other government initiatives aimed at 'measuring what counts', incorporating performance targets, benchmarking of performance and publication of comparative metrics. Patients were reframed as consumers and rational 'choosers' of health services, whilst the responsibility for purchasing and maintaining IT systems – which enabled the measurement procedures – shifted away from GPs to the (now disbanded) Primary Care Organisations. IT systems had to be accredited against UK-wide standards and became essential to the delivery of QOF. Ostensibly QOF was introduced as a 'voluntary' incentive scheme designed to encourage practices to attain clearly defined quality standards, but by the time of my data collection QOF constituted about 30 per cent of practice remuneration. Critics argued that 'what starts as an incentive becomes coercion when it represents such a large proportion of practice income that its loss becomes a credible threat' (Mangin and Toop, 2007). QOF was a significant driver in bringing the EPR centre stage in general practice. Once in place this has opened up scope for many measurement and surveillance activities by external bodies. QOF is one example of an external institutional 'voice' which the EPR delivers directly into the consultation.

Chronic disease management consultations often open with a scoping statement such as 'How have things been from the diabetes point of view?'; 'We want to look at things from the cardiac point of view' or the shorter version 'So ... asthma review'. Consultations typically start and finish with the same questions and there is a clear focus on data gathering and documentation. Nurses have to work hard to avoid privileging 'institution-centred' care over 'patient-centred' care and vary in their capacity to achieve this. It takes considerable creativity to sustain the projection of professional 'self' as involved primarily with the patient and their unique circumstances in this environment. When nurses manage this well, any evidence of this creative work becomes invisible in the resulting documentation as flexible creativity is not part of the inflexible 'model' which informs the template's design. This is a persistent challenge of computerised work in which some practices become increasingly visible and open to surveillance, whilst other forms of expertise fall into the shadows (Star and Strauss, 1999). Patients with a chronic disease all start to look the same, as do the clinicians caring for them. What is unique and individual is an ephemeral feature of the consultation as the 'selves' of both patient and nurse become marginalised in the institutional account. A reader of the completed template would struggle to find what is unique and individual to the patient's narrative. Patients' stories morph into bytes of data, the particular becomes generalised, the complex is made discrete, simple and manageable and uncertainty becomes categorised as certainty and 'contained' (Swinglehurst *et al.*, 2012).

Here is a shortened version of field notes which I made during and after observing a nurse's coronary heart disease clinic (see also Swinglehurst, 2015).

Field notes of a computer crash

We were between patients when the computer crashed. The nurse rushed into the corridor to be met by a secretary who was panicking because the usual IT person was on holiday. I followed the secretary downstairs.

The tiny office next to reception was soon full. The secretary talked to the IT supplier on the phone and two of the GPs knelt on the floor round the server, bums in the air, fiddling with buttons, while an alarm sounded. Another GP joked from the side-lines about the reliability of IT. One of the receptionists asked me: 'Does this never happen in your place?' Patients kept arriving but the receptionists didn't know who to expect. The waiting room was filling up.

After a few minutes, some lights flashed on the server and there was a collective sigh of relief amongst the GPs, who returned to their rooms to resume clinic.

I went back to the nurse's room. She was flustered as she went downstairs to find her next patient. As they returned I heard her warning: 'We've got a problem 'cos the computer isn't working'.

They sat down. The nurse said 'I'll have to do it a little out of order because I've no computer'.

Like many consultations I had observed the nurse asked: 'Do you know which medicines you are on, from a <u>cardiac</u> point of view?' This use of this phrase 'cardiac point of view' was familiar. On this occasion I couldn't help noticing that for the first time it was the patient rather than the computer screen to whom it was directed. The patient took a list of drugs from her handbag and gave it to the nurse saying, 'I'm prepared for all eventualities, my dear'.

The nurse struggled to identify what to do next. She kept checking and rechecking the blank computer screen, and made comments such as, 'This is *so* confusing not having the computer.'

After a brief return of computer activity, it crashed again, prompting the nurse to say, 'Sadly our return to the computer was only temporary, so I can't do anything at the moment.'

Part way through this somewhat chaotic consultation she apologised saying, 'I'm sorry it's been such a higgledy-piggledy consultation.' She left the consulting room twice, on one occasion saying she was going to find out if she was the only one still having computer problems.

At the close of the consultation the nurse apologised again 'I'm sorry. It was a bit of a come and go consultation,' to which the patient replied 'WELL DONE,' then added gently '... you can go off computers.'

The unexpected disruption made this consultation difficult. This is understandable, especially in the context that a researcher is observing. The extract illustrates some of the ways in which professional clinical practice is shaped and 'ordered' by the EPR.

First, the nurse's comments point to a sense that the consultation *should* be an orderly affair guided by the fields in the computer template ('I'll have to do it a little out of order'; 'I'm sorry it was such a higgledy-piggledy consultation'). Perhaps the most striking observation is the extent to which the nurse's moment-by-moment conduct in the consultation has become interwoven with using the technology. The nurse is senior, popular, well-liked and more than capable of conducting a routine cardiovascular check without the electronic prompts. But it seems that her embodied practices have become so finely tuned to incorporate the template that to 'go on' without it has become almost impossible. The nurse uses a rhetorical device called an extreme case formulation (Pomerantz, 1986) as a way of emphasising this difficulty ('I can't do anything at the moment'). The performance of 'self' is an embodied one, shaped in part through interactions with human beings but also through interactions with material artefacts (such as the list of medicines pulled from the patient's handbag in response to a question) and technologies. Both nurse and patient have to improvise in the circumstances in order find alternative ways to 'go on' and both engage in face-work. For example, the nurse warns the patient of the computer problem in advance ('we've got a problem') paving the way for a consultation which she anticipates may not go as smoothly as it might under usual circumstances; the patient congratulates the nurse for managing despite this ('well done') and her list of medicines is a useful stand-in for the computer (and serves as an answer to a question that she may or may not know the answer to). Between them they make it to the end of the consultation, relationship intact. They share a sense of agreement that the consultation was not entirely satisfactory, but both agree that the 'problem' was not of their own making ('you can go off computers').

One challenge of the chronic disease clinic is that the purpose of the clinic is 'disease specific' but the patients attending, like Edith, often have many medical problems. This fragmentation of the 'self' (first the separation of the disease from the person or 'self' who has the disease, then also the separation into *different* diseases for different occasions of care) is problematic. Take this example:

Multimorbidity in the single disease clinic

A frail 86-year-old man struggled in to the clinic, barely able to walk. He was very deaf. He hung his walking stick over the chair and grimaced as he sat down, looking as if he was in pain.

The nurse said loudly: 'We've called you in to look at you from the heart point of view. I know you have a lot of other things going on but we've called you in to look at your heart.' She then asked, 'How often do you use the angina tablet under your tongue?'

The patient replied in a way which made his most pressing concern clear: 'Not much … for the simple reason that I can only crawl like a tortoise.'

Nurse: 'And the simvastatin?'

Patient: 'No … I stopped that. I think it's giving me diarrhoea. These hearing aids are not very good you know. I've had it adjusted several times but I'm really disappointed. I had hoped for better than this'.

The nurse's comment 'I know you have a lot of other things going on, but we've called you in to look at your heart' serves several functions. She explicitly acknowledges the difficulty inherent in fragmenting the 'self' and narrowing the focus onto the heart problem when the patient has a 'lot of other things going on'. In doing this she conveys a sense of 'knowing the patient as a whole person' – a performance of face-work in which she presents her 'self' as the kind of nurse who cares about this wider experience.

There is then a 'scale jump' (Blommaert, 2006), meaning that the nurse moves quickly from this individual unique 'here and now' framing ('I know you have') to a more general institutional framing ('we've called you in'). This shift is effective in making plain what Goodwin calls 'figure' (your heart) and 'ground' (the rest) (Goodwin, 1994), setting out what is more and less relevant. The shift from 'I know' to 'we've called' also saves the nurse's face by distancing her personally from the institutional procedure of recall (in this instance it is clear that the patient has endured a struggle to attend).

The patient uses simile ('like a tortoise') and an abrupt change in footing in his final utterance to steer attention towards his prime concerns of poor mobility and deafness. These are not pursued any further, nor are they documented. That his mobility is so poor that his angina is barely triggered is an unremarkable problem in this clinic. This is not so much about there being no field for these in the template. Rather that the practice of using a template shapes up how disease, illness and the 'self' are made sense of in the clinic (Swinglehurst *et al.*, 2012). They offer neither patient nor nurse much space for consideration of unanticipated contingencies, uncertainties, alternative logics, emotional work or less fragmented all-encompassing notions of 'selfhood'. I will summarise this as the disturbing scarcity of simple questions such as 'How are *you*?' or 'How have *you* been?'

Creative work with templates

In their work with templates, clinicians maintain a dual orientation towards providing individual patient care and gathering institutional data (such as QOF data) in the form of standard codes. The latter are often difficult to tease out and negotiate. There are also demands to re-contextualise the 'particular' into more 'general' terms. Just as moral work is invoked whenever we are called to apply a general rule to a particular case (e.g. a national guideline for an individual patient), moral work is also involved when we derive a general account from the particular experience. I will illustrate this by reference to another example, this time from the asthma clinic.

Tom had booked to see a nurse in the asthma clinic when he turned up at the reception desk to request an inhaler from his repeat medication list. The receptionist noticed a reminder in his EPR that his asthma review was now due. Tom had run out of inhalers after a particularly difficult episode of being awake all night with asthma symptoms.

At the beginning of the consultation the nurse skilfully elicits the patient's story, jotting some notes on paper, and establishes that Tom does not understand how to use his inhalers. She spends a long time working carefully with Tom to help him understand how to manage his asthma symptoms. She turns to the computer to complete the EPR template, arriving at a set of prompts about asthma symptoms, including one which asks her to document whether asthma is disturbing sleep ('A: disturbing sleep' or 'B: not disturbing sleep'). This prompts the nurse to revisit this issue again (see Figure 3.2).

Given what we know already about Tom and the circumstances of this consultation we might expect the nurse to pass over this quickly (by selecting

Time		Words	Bodily conduct
12:07	N	And do:: you	N <->P
		(0.2)	
		uhm I know recently the other n- n:ight you said you	N points to paper on her desk
		woke up during the night	
	P	=mm=	P <-> N; P nods head
12:12	N	= with:: breathlessness	P <-> N
		(0.4)	
12:14	N	Is that something that occurs regularly.	
		(1.0)	
12:17	P	Uhm	P shifts around in chair, looks ahead. N looking at P.
		(0.2)	
		its occurred a coup- uh bout a couple of times but not	P returns gaze to N
		>sort of< =	
12:20	N	= a couple of times in the past how long	P <->N
		(1.8)	P <-> N
	P	°how long°	P <-> N
		what how long ago::	N leans back in chair, maintaining gaze with P
12:25	N	YEH (.)	
		you say a couple of times what	N puts both hands parallel in between N and P
		>a couple of times< in the last ye::ar	N makes emphatic arm movements, shifting parallel hands to her far left, and downward marking on "year"
		>a couple of times< in the last mo::nth?	N – similar arm movement, with downward marking on "month" but just left of centre, maintaining gaze on P
		(0.2)	N puts hands together centrally
12:30	P	°>A couple of times< in the last year°	P <-> N
12:31	N	A couple of times in the last year so that's fine, so its not (.) regularly.	N nods and turns head to face EPR, body part way between two. P looks at keyboard. N keeps L arm on arm of her chair so partially oriented towards P
12:35	P	no=	P shakes head
	N	=((C))	N types keystroke
		°°occurring°°	P shakes head, sits forward and turns to look at EPRv

Figure 3.2 Nurse establishing whether the patient's asthma is disturbing sleep.

A: disturbing sleep). But the nurse's task is to establish whether this occurs *regularly;* she is seeking a more general account.

She restarts her first utterance at 12:07 with some repair work. To complete the question (e.g. Do you have sleep disturbance? or Do you wake at night?) would suggest failure to listen earlier in the consultation and threaten loss of face. There is a long pause and Tom wriggles in his chair before offering a hesitant reply, which the nurse interrupts in order to seek clarity on the notion of 'regularity'. A misunderstanding occurs at 12:20; the patient does not follow what the nurse means by '<u>how</u> long'. The nurse suggests two possible time-frames and uses elaborate hand gestures to enhance the explanation.

Although the patient is not limited to these two options, this way of phrasing the question does encourage selection of one of them. Tom responds in a hushed voice, choosing the first option ('A couple of times in the last year'), appropriating the nurse's words as his own (Bakhtin, 1981b). In this agreement, he actively saves the face of the nurse and keeps the interaction on track. The phrase 'couple of times' features seven times in this short extract as participants re-appropriate each other's words as their own.

If we ask Bakhtin's question 'Who is doing the talking?' at 12.30 the answer is not straightforward. It is certainly not convincing that Tom is committed to these words as an account of his *actual* experience. The nurse responds 'A couple of times in the last year so that's fine. So it's not ... regularly.' As she turns to the EPR to select response 'B' (i.e. not disturbing sleep), the topic is closed.

This short exchange shows face-work in action as both nurse and patient orient to the institutional work that needs to be done to complete the template whilst working hard to maintain the flow of the communication and maintain a consistent (and cooperative) image of their 'selves' in their roles of nurse and patient. The use of the EPR template prompts recycling of the topic and we see how the moral work of 'squeezing' the particular story into a generalised account plays out in practice. When templates are used elastic concepts and rich personal narratives are moulded into binary constructs; Tom's particular story of being awake all night with asthma symptoms vanishes in the generalised institutional account. It takes a lot of interactive work to 'succeed' in weaving a relatively bureaucratic process into a personal encounter (Checkland *et al.*, 2007; Roberts and Campbell, 2005) and the resulting template is always an 'incomplete' compromise. In this example we see two challenges to the self. First there is the marginalisation of the personal narrative in the documentation. At the same time the template generates a new kind of work that is socially very demanding of the 'self' as the nurse negotiates with the patient how to achieve this documentation.

One nurse described herself as being a 'paper person' but also used the words 'template driven' to describe her approach in the diabetes clinic. She had negotiated longer appointments with her employers (now 30 minutes instead of 15) so she could retain what she regarded as a 'patient-centred' approach 'otherwise I would have just been completing the boxes with no time for the patient'. Her words suggest that 'completing the boxes' sits uncomfortably with being '*for* the patient'. This nurse went to great lengths to minimise time spent facing the computer, seizing opportunities to do so as patients were removing socks or tying shoelaces. She went into clinic 30 minutes early. During this time she meticulously studied the EPR of each patient she was due to see, copying blood results and other information she thought she may need to refer to later in the consultation. When consulting, she often placed her left hand on the patient's arm as she rotated her chair towards the EPR screen, keeping it there as she typed with her right hand. This was an awkward posture, but it allowed her to maintain a physical connection to the patient as she attended to the EPR.

Watching her in clinic, I came to realise that she 'knew' the template and had internalised it. She worked *with it* in a semiotic sense and wove it skilfully into the consultation but kept it relatively invisible to patients, marginalising it from her embodied activity. Her performed self was as a 'paper person' who preferred to be *for* the patient in this template-oriented world. She was also 'template driven' in that she took seriously the requirement to complete the template – but she was also 'driven' to find creative ways of working around it. It had become part of a new professional 'self'. This was costly. The nurse managed the tension between person-centred care and the needs of the institution but this came with an opportunity cost to herself in terms of time, and a financial cost to her employer (her consultations were now twice as long).

Examples of such creativity stood out as examples of what Blommaert has called *creativity within constraints* (Blommaert, 2005a, p. 207) noticeable because it creates understandable contrasts to normative standards.

Now my computer's asked me...

The EPR is awash with prompts, alerts and reminders. For example it displays alerts showing which QOF data are missing from the patient's record. These prompts may be tangential to the current consultation but serve as a constant reminder of institutional imperatives and of a tension between the need to attend to the patient's immediate concerns and those demanded by institutions such as the Clinical Commissioning Group or NHS ('dilemma of attention').

This is troublesome. Such reminders are not neutral since they come to define what is regarded as important 'knowledge' about patients and, in the case of QOF constitute definitions of 'quality' in practice (Swinglehurst, 2014). The moral question of 'whose interests to serve' becomes particularly salient in a consultation which is already constrained by pressures of time. As one GP said 'If they want me to collect brownie points then I can ... but the patients are being robbed of their consultation'. The decision to ignore or bypass a prompt that is aligned institutionally with notions of 'quality' in practice is a difficult one, since by implication it suggests that this is the kind of activity a 'quality' clinician will do. The challenge is not simply one of attending to additional topics, but managing the additional complexity of interactional work that arises from having to account for this 'institutional' activity in the personal encounter with the patient.

I will illustrate this with another example. At the time of my data collection doctors were required to document whether patients over 15 were smokers or non-smokers. Figure 3.3 shows an extract from a consultation when the GP attends to one of these prompts (QOF: Recent Smoking Data). The GP has already addressed the patient's gynaecological problem, examined the patient and arranged a referral. The prompt has been displayed on the screen throughout the consultation.

The first thing to note is the doctor pointing to the EPR screen as she announces 'now my computer's asked me whether you smoke'. The doctor enacts a change in footing, with the contextualisation cue 'now' and her pointing. The patient joins the doctor in looking at the screen and hesitates, offering a non-committal response 'yes ... no'. In suggesting it is the computer which has 'asked' the question, the doctor attributes it partial agency and introduces some 'attributional distance' between herself and the question that she is asking (Clayman, 1992) thus marking it out as a delicate matter. The doctor makes it clear to the patient that she is responding to a wider institutional voice. The categorisation work (smoker or non-smoker) is not straightforward, but the doctor (like the nurse in Figure 3.2) presses on to try to assign a value to the number of

Time	D P	Words spoken /sounds	Bodily conduct	EPR Screen
14.32	D	now my computer's	D - > EPR. D points to screen	Medications screen.
		asked me whether you smoke	D - > EPR, L hand to mouth; P –> EPR;	QOF alert showing in bottom R corner: QOF Recent Smoking Data (displays throughout consultation)
		(1.2)	D - > P; P - > EPR	
14.35	P	uhm	P - > EPR	
		(1.0)		
14.36	P	yes (.) no	P - > EPR; D - > P	
		(1.0)	P - > D	
14.38	D	he what's [that mean	D - > EPR, laughing	
	P	[I've had _one_ in the last three days	D < -> P	
14.41	D	right (.) so (.) very occasionally	D < -> P	
14.43	P	yeah (0.2) I'm (.) I'm very much a s:ocial smoker nowadays=		
	D	= so with- in a (0.2) in a week uhm how many do you get through °d'you think°		
14.49	P	well last week I think I had three		
14.52	D	right (0.4) right		
		(5.0)	D turns - > EPR; P - > D. At 14.57 D turns to P again	
Transcript not shown – doctor establishes that patient smoked three cigarettes last week and suggests it would be better for patient's general health if she could 'ignore them', since although it is not doing 'horrendous damage' it is still keeping the 'receptors flapping'				
15.29	D	so (0.2) y'know obviously	D - > EPR; P - > D	
		°<as your _doctor_ > I have to advise you that you shouldn't°	D < - > P; D using highly stylised voice	
		(1.6)	D nods, smiling	

Figure 3.3 GP responding to an EPR prompt.

cigarettes the patient smokes 'in general'. Traditionally, medical records have been a source of information about what is known about the patient, but here it is not what known but what is *not* known and *ought to be known* which comes to the foreground (the deontic voice of the EPR, actively shaping what *should* be done).

Although the consultation has always presented the possibility of opportunistic health promotion advice (it features in Stott and Davies' model of the consultation) (Stott and Davis, 1979) the use of the EPR as a prompt to this kind of talk encompasses a shift for the doctor from the 'professional' self towards an emphasis on institutional evidence and accountability. We see the interactional work that the doctor does to navigate this transition at 15.29: 'so (0.2) y'know obviously < as your doctor > I have to advise you that you shouldn't'. She enacts an obvious change in footing through various means. First, she slows down and quietens her speech markedly ('< as your doctor >') deliberately drawing attention to being active in a professional capacity. She then uses a highly stylised voice as she continues: 'I have to advise you that you shouldn't'.

This is 'hybrid discourse' (Roberts *et al.*, 2000; Sarangi and Roberts, 1999) in that it is legitimate professional advice on the one hand but it also orients to a higher 'institutional' order or institutional imperative, incorporating an element of *accounting* for this professional talk. The use of 'I have to' both points to this institutional imperative and also creates attributional distance as the doctor performs a 'new' self as institutional representative. Like the nurses described above, the doctor makes the role of the EPR in guiding her actions explicit, but then has to be creative in managing the transition between her projected professional 'self' and her parallel role as institutional representative.

Conclusions

Across many of the examples in this chapter we see how the EPR profoundly shapes the consultation and is integral to the social practices in the consulting room. It is not simply a 'data container' but presents a range of new opportunities and new demands; it also creates new forms of order and new 'work'. This new work is a challenge to the performance of the professional 'self' since the EPR encourages a certain direction of travel – tending to shift towards a privileging of the 'institutional' version of the patient over the patient as 'individual' or sharpening the tension between institution-centred care (bringing with it additional surveillance and accountability) over patient-centred care.

We have also seen the determined efforts of clinicians working persistently, moment-by-moment, to counter this tendency and maintain a coherent sense of professional self in this challenging context. This construction of self occurs in the small details of talk and bodily conduct, and arises through social interaction. The EPR *shapes* but doesn't *make*; it *constrains* but does not *prohibit*; it *makes possible* but does not necessarily *insist*. The social impact of the EPR on the 'selves' of patient and clinician is at the same time *profound* and yet *provisional* and depends on the immediate social context of its actual use in practice.

I am drawn to the words of Erickson which seem particularly fitting when we consider the highly creative and improvisatory work that professionals do to keep their consultations 'on track', smooth things over and maintain good relationships with patients in the face of such challenges to the 'self'. On each occasion of using the EPR, they work through local contingencies and there is always some room for creativity. It is in this local creativity that there is reason for optimism in what can otherwise appear a rather gloomy picture of technocratic rule.

> The agency manifested by local social actors in bricolage and improvisation can be employed either counter-hegemonically or hegemonically, regressively or progressively, despicably or admirably. One can swim downstream with the prevailing currents of social structuration and history, treating as limits the constraints one encounters, or one can swim upstream, treating the prestructured constraints as affordances for maneuvering towards ends other than those that are societally approved or expected. The latter course costs more in terms of effort, and it risks punishment. But it is possible.
>
> (Erickson, 2004, p. 174)

Key learning points

- Close consideration of the dynamics of the consultation offer insights into the performance and construction of the 'self-hood'.
- The 'self' is constructed moment-by-moment as participants in the consultation contribute to (and respond to) the ongoing social context in a sophisticated and highly nuanced way.
- Technologies such as the EPR profoundly shape and challenge the dynamics of the clinical consultation and are integral to this social context in the contemporary consultation.
- The EPR introduces new 'voices' into the consultation. Clinicians adopt a range of strategies to weave these voices into the consultation whilst maintaining a coherent presentation of 'self'. This is demanding work, especially when the unique needs of the patient compete with the needs of the wider institution for standardised data.

Notes

1 The transcribing conventions for the data extracts presented in this chapter are based on Atkinson and Heritage (1984) and can be found in the Appendix on p. 169.
2 The authorship of some of the Bakhtin/Vološinov writings is controversial, with some critics believing that work attributed to Vološinov may actually have been written by Bakhtin. For the purpose of this chapter Bakhtinian refers to the work of Bakhtin and/ or Vološinov.

74   D. Swinglehurst

References

Atkinson, J.M. and Heritage, J. 1984. Transcript notation. *In:* J.M. Atkinson and J. Heritage (eds) *Structures of social action: studies in conversation analysis* (p. ix–xvi). Cambridge: Cambridge University Press.

Bakhtin, M. 1981a. Discourse in the Novel. *In:* Holquist, M. (ed.) *The dialogic imagination: four essays by M.M. Bakhtin.* Austin: University of Texas Press.

Bakhtin, M. 1981b. *The dialogic imagination: four essays.* Texas: University of Texas Press.

Balint, M. 1964. *The doctor, his patient and the illness.* Edinburgh: Churchill Livingstone.

Berg, M. 1996. Practices or reading and writing: the constitutive role of the patient record in medical work. *Sociology of Health and Illness*, 18: 499–524.

Berg, M. 1997. Of Forms, Containers, and the Electronic Medical Record: Some Tools for a Sociology of the Formal. *Science, Technology and Human Values*, 22: 403–33.

Berg, M. 1998. Medical work and the computer-based patient record: a sociological perspective. *Methods Inf.Med.*, 37: 294–301.

Berg, M. 2004. Health care work and patient care information systems. *Health Information Management – integrating information technology in health care work.*

Berger, J. and Mohr, J. 1967. *A fortunate man; the story of a country doctor.* London: The Penguin Press.

Blommaert, J. 2005a. *Discourse.* Cambridge: Cambridge University Press.

Blommaert, J. 2005b. Text and context. *Discourse.* Cambridge: Cambridge University Press.

Blommaert, J. 2006. Sociolinguistic scales. *Working Papers in Urban Language and Literacies, Paper 37.* Institute of Education.

Casey, M., Shaw, S. and Swinglehurst, D. 2017. Online consultation systems: case study of experiences in one early adopter site. *BJGP*, in press.

Charon, R. 2001. Narrative Medicine: Form, Function, and Ethics. *Annals of Internal Medicine*, 134: 83–7.

Checkland, K., McDonald, R. and Harrison, S. 2007. Ticking Boxes and Changing the Social World: Data Collection and the New UK General Practice Contract. *Social Policy and Administration*, 41: 693–710.

Clayman, S.E. 1992. Footing in the achievement of neutrality: the case of news-interview discourse. *In:* Drew, P. and Heritage, J. (eds) *Talk at Work: Interaction in institutional settings.* Cambridge: Cambridge University Press.

Creese, A. 2008. Linguistic Ethnography. *In:* King, K.A. and Hornberger, N.H. (eds) *Encyclopedia of language and education.* New York: Springer Science and Business Media LLC.

Erickson, F. 2004. *Talk and social theory.* Cambridge: Polity.

Erickson, F. and Shultz, J. 1982. Aspects of Social Organisation in Communicative Performance. *In: The counselor as gatekeeper.* New York, London: Academic Press.

Goffman, E. 1959. *The presentation of self in everyday life.* New York: Doubleday Anchor.

Goffman, E. 1966. Involvement. *In: Behavior in public places.* New York: The Free Press.

Goffman, E. 1967. On Face-work. *In: Interaction ritual: essays on face-to-face behaviour.* New York: Pantheon Books.

Goffman, E. 1981. Footing. *In: Forms of talk.* Philadelphia: University of Pennsylvania Press.

Goodwin, C. 1994. Professional Vision. *American Anthropologist*, 96: 606–33.

Greatbatch, D. 1992. *System Use and Interpersonal Communication in the General Practice Consultation: Preliminary Observations.* Cambridge: Rank Xerox Research Centre.

Greatbatch, D., Heath, C., Campion, P. and Luff, P. 1995. How do desk-top computers affect the doctor-patient interaction? *Family Practice*, 12: 32–6.

Greatbatch, D., Luff, P., Heath, C. and Campion, P. 1993. Interpersonal communication and human-computer interaction: an examination of the use of computers in medical consultations. *Interacting with Computers*, 5: 193–216.

Greenhalgh, T. and Hurwitz, B. 1999. Why study narrative? *BMJ*, 318, 48–50.

Greenhalgh, T., Potts, H.W.W., Wong, G., Bark, P. and Swinglehurst, D. 2009. Tensions and Paradoxes in Electronic Patient Record Research: A Systematic Literature Review Using the Meta-narrative Method. *The Milbank Quarterly*, 87: 729–88.

Gumperz, J.J. 1982. Contextualising conventions. *In:* Gumperz, J.J. (ed.) *Discourse strategies.* Cambridge: Cambridge University Press.

Gumperz, J.J. 1992. Contextualisation and understanding. *In:* Duranti, A. and Goodwin, C. (eds) *Rethinking context.* Cambridge: Cambridge University Press.

Harrison, S. 2002. New Labour, Modernisation and the Medical Labour Process. *Journal of Social Policy*, 31: 465–85.

Heath, I. 1995. *The Mystery of General Practice.* London: Nuffield Provincial Hospitals Trust.

Heeks, R., Mundy, D. and Salazar, A. 1999. *Why health care information systems succeed or fail. Information Systems for Public Sector Management Working Paper Series.* Institute for Development Policy and Management, University of Manchester. Available at: www.sed.manchester.ac.uk/idpm/publications/wp/igov/igov_wp09.pdf

Heritage, J. 2001. Goffman, Garfinkel and Conversation Analysis. *In:* Wetherell, M., Taylor, S. and Yates, S. (eds) *Discourse theory and practice.* London: Sage Publications.

Julian, P. 1987. Being there. *In:* Elder, A. and Samuel, O. (eds) *While I'm here, doctor.* London: Tavistock/Routledge.

Kumarapeli, P. and De Lusignan, S. 2013. Using the computer in the clinical consultation; setting the stage, reviewing, recording, and taking actions: a multi-channel video study. *Journal of the American Medical Informatics Association*, 20: e67–e75.

Mangin, D. and Toop, L. 2007. The Quality and Outcomes Framework: what have you done to yourselves? *British Journal of General Practice*, 57: 435–7.

May, C., Rapley, T., Moreira, T., Finch, T. and Heaven, B. 2006. Technogovernance: Evidence, subjectivity, and the clinical encounter in primary care medicine. *Social Science and Medicine*, 62: 1022–30.

Maybin, J. 2001. Language, Struggle and Voice: The Bakhtin/Vološinov Writings. *In:* Wetherell, M., Taylor, S. and Yates, S. (eds) *Discourse theory and practice.* London: Sage Publications.

NHS England 2016. *General practice forward view.*

Oesterlund, C. 2002. *Documenting dreams: patient-centred records versus practice-centred records.* Doctor of Philosophy in Management, Massachusetts Institute of Technology.

Pearce, C. 2007. *Doctors, patients and computers, the new consultation.* PhD thesis, Department of General Practice, The University of Melbourne.

Pearce, C., Dwan, K., Arnold, M., Phillips, C. and Trumble, S. 2009. Doctor, patient and computer – a framework for the new consultation. *International Journal of Medical Informatics*, 78: 32–8.

Pearce, C., Trumble, S., Arnold, M., Dwan, K. and Phillips, C. 2008. Computers in the new consultation: within the first minute. *Family Practice*, 25: 202–8.

Polanyi, M. 1958. *Personal knowledge: towards a post-critical philosophy*. Chicago: The University of Chicago Press.

Pomerantz, A. 1986. Extreme case formulations: a new way of legitimating claims. *Human Studies (Interaction and Language Use Special Issue)*, 9: 219–30.

Rampton, B. 2007. *Linguistic ethnography and the study of identities.* King's College London. Available at: www.kcl.ac.uk/innovation/groups/ldc/publications/working papers/43.pdf

Roberts, C. and Campbell, S. 2005. Fitting stories into boxes: rhetorical and textual constraints on candidates' performances in British job interviews. *Journal of Applied Linguistics*, 2: 45–73.

Roberts, C. and Sarangi, S. 2005. Theme-oriented discourse analysis of medical encounters. *Medical Education*, 39: 632–40.

Roberts, C., Sarangi, S., Southgate, L., Wakeford, R. and Wass, V. 2000. Oral examination – equal opportunities, ethnicity, and fairness in the MRCGP. *BMJ*, 320: 370–5.

Sarangi, S. and Roberts, C. 1999. The dynamics of interactional and institutional orders in work-related settings. *In:* Sarangi, S. and Roberts, C. (eds) *Talk, work and institutional order.* Berlin, New York: Mouton de Gruyter.

Schön, D.A. 1983. *The reflective practitioner: how professionals think in action.* New York: Basic Books Inc.

Scott, D. and Purves, I. 1996. Triadic relationship between doctor, computer and patient. *Interacting with Computers*, 8: 347–63.

Snell, J.E., Shaw, S.E. and Copland, F.E. 2015. *Linguistic ethnography: interdisciplinary explorations.* Basingstoke: Palgrave Macmillan.

Star, S.L. and Strauss, A. 1999. Layers of silence, arenas of voice: The ecology of visible and invisible work. *Computer supported cooperative work (CSCW)*, 8: 9–30.

Stott, N.C.H. and Davis, R.H. 1979. The Exceptional Potential in each Primary Care Consultation. *Journal of the Royal College of General Practitioners*, 29: 201–5.

Swinglehurst, D. 2014. Displays of authority in the clinical consultation: a linguistic ethnographic study of the electronic patient record. *Soc Sci Med*, 118: 17–26.

Swinglehurst, D. 2015. How linguistic ethnography may enhance our understanding of electronic patient records in healthcare settings (in press). *In:* Snell, F., Shaw, S.E. and Copland, F. (eds) *Linguistic ethnography: interdisciplinary explorations.* London: Palgrave Macmillan.

Swinglehurst, D. and Greenhalgh, T. 2015. Caring for the patient, caring for the record: an ethnographic study of 'back office' work in upholding quality of care in general practice. *BMC Health Serv Res*, 15: 177.

Swinglehurst, D., Greenhalgh, T. and Roberts, C. 2012. Computer templates in chronic disease management: ethnographic case study in general practice. *BMJ Open*, 2:e001754, doi: 10.1136/bmjopen-2012-001754.

Swinglehurst, D., Roberts, C. and Greenhalgh, T. 2011. Opening Up the 'Black Box' of the Electronic Patient Record: A Linguistic Ethnographic Study in General Practice. *Communication and Medicine*, 8.

Toon, P.D.A. 2014. *A flourishing practice?* London: RCGP.

Vološinov, V. 1973. *Marxism and the philosophy of language*, Cambridge, MA: Harvard University Press.

4   Subjectivity of patients and doctors

Iona Heath

Orientation

My principal expertise is as a clinician and, in particular, as a generalist clinician. From that perspective, I have found biomedical science of very little help in my efforts to understand the experience of subjectivity or what is meant by the self. I have learnt much more from my observation of, and participation within, the activities of clinical practice and even more from refracting these lessons through the lenses of literature, history, politics and, to a lesser extent, anthropology. However the reader should be aware that I am an expert in none of these marvellous humanistic disciplines.

My pragmatic working definition is that the self is the recipient and the holder of all subjective experience built up in stories and memories over a lifetime, and an agent with at least some ability to shape and influence that experience. It is the self which renders every single human being, alive or dead, unlike any other. Each self is created and either thrives or struggles within a web of human relationships and each of these webs in also unique. It is the individual self within its contextual web which becomes the object of healthcare. Yet, as we saw in Chapter 1, as healthcare systems have become increasingly industrialised, bureaucratised and standardised over the last 50 years, there has been a worsening tendency for the individuality and subjectivity of both patients and doctors to be marginalised. Patients have been reduced to standardised units of healthcare need whose predicament can be encapsulated within a computer code and resolved through the application of an algorithm (Holmes, 2014), while doctors and other healthcare professionals are reduced to units of healthcare provision whose activities are powerfully constrained by guidelines, targets and financial incentives (McKee and Clarke, 1995). Worse still, the continuing relationship between a patient self and a doctor self has come to be regarded as unimportant. Medical science has made huge strides in understanding the biology of the human body while, at the same time, clinical practice has regressed through the neglect of the subjective experience of both patients and doctors. As American philosopher Martha Nussbaum writes:

> each of the strategies used to make practical wisdom more scientific and more in control ... leads to a distinct impoverishment of the world of practice.
>
> (Nussbaum, 1986)

Totalitarianism and the self

I will start with history and politics as it is the global political context of rampant neoliberal capitalism that has driven the industrialisation of medical care and the legitimation of the pursuit of financial profit (McGregor, 2001). The sociologist Zygmunt Bauman describes the invasive and parasitical nature of neoliberalism which drives:

> the shift from the 'society of producers' to the 'society of consumers', and from the meeting of capital and labour to the meeting of commodity and client as the principal source of 'added value' … substituting desire for need in the role of the fly-wheel of the profit-aimed economy.
>
> (Bauman, 2011)

These are the processes that are distorting healthcare and, because efficient markets require standardised products, have systematically marginalised the importance of subjectivity and the self.

In this context, we need to take seriously the warning that, if we cannot remember the past, we are condemned to repeat it (Santayana, 1980). Political totalitarianism demands the complete subservience of the individual to the state and I am going to argue that the subservience of the self within contemporary healthcare systems threatens to create a form of social totalitarianism. George Steiner recognises the tendency of totalitarianism to demand the suppression of memory – both individual and collective:

> Soviet totalitarianism is most extreme not in the claims it makes on the utopian future, but in the violence it would do to the past, to the vital integrity of human remembrance.
>
> (Steiner, 1967)

Similarly, in his essay on Virgil published in 1944, T.S. Eliot writes about history, the loss of memory and a new provincialism of time:

> In our age, when men seem … to try to solve problems of life in terms of engineering, there is coming into existence a new kind of provincialism which perhaps deserves a new name. It is a provincialism, not of space, but of time; one for which history is merely the chronicle of human devices which have served their turn and been scrapped, one for which the world is the property solely of the living, a property in which the dead hold no shares.
>
> (Eliot, 1945)

Contemporary healthcare is deeply enmeshed in this new kind of provincialism. Medicine has an obsession with scientific progress and a misplaced belief in the perfectibility of the human body and mind and, as a result, there seems never to be time for the necessary backward glance. In order to resist this damaging trend, I intend to invoke thinkers and writers who lived lives scarred by totalitarian politics. If we are to learn any of the lessons of history, and restore subjectivity and selfhood to the centre of healthcare, we need to learn from those who have suffered at the sharp end of political totalitarianism and who have subsequently thought deeply about the implications of their experience.

The political philosopher Karl Popper who was born in Austria in 1902 was baptised a Lutheran, but was of Jewish heritage. Fearing the rise of Nazism, he left Austria before the 1938 Anschluss, going first to Christchurch in New Zealand and then to London. In 1945, Popper published *The Open Society and Its Enemies* which is his response to the rise of totalitarianism and the perhaps his most famous book. He argued that there is a danger of totalitarianism whenever an abstract concept is allowed to trump the needs of actual living persons, as when the needs of some collective social entity (be it, for example, a city, a state, society, a nation, a race, or even a healthcare system) is found to have needs that are prior and superior to the needs of actual living persons. The selfhood that we are trying to recover belongs to Popper's actual living persons and so we need to be concerned whenever the self is ignored, marginalised or downgraded in importance.

Popper described two contrasting approaches to social reform. The first is utopian social engineering which is motivated by a vision of what a perfect society would look like and which seeks to achieve this by whatever means available. This becomes a solution imposed by its creators and although intentions are often admirable, they are pervaded by the false certainty and the all-too-common conviction of knowing what is good for other people and knowing how other people should live their lives, which seems so prevalent within contemporary healthcare. In contrast, Popper favoured the second approach of piecemeal engineering which concentrates on the most pressing existing social problems and proceeds incrementally. All experience tells us that change always produces unintended as well as intended consequences. With piecemeal engineering, incremental iterative change makes it easier to identify and mitigate the unintended consequences. According to Popper, utopian engineering aims at a perfect state and therefore requires centralised control which lapses all too easily into dictatorship. He summarised his position in one memorable sentence:

The attempt to make heaven on earth invariably produces hell.

(Popper, 1945)

George Katkov was Popper's contemporary and fellow philosopher, and similarly, a political refugee to Britain. He was born in Moscow in 1903, lived through the Russian Revolution, but was living in Prague by 1929 where he got his PhD and escaped to Britain days before the outbreak of the Second World War.

In 1951, by then living in England, Katkov invoked the careless calculus of the utilitarianism promulgated by Jeremy Bentham:

It is the greatest happiness of the greatest number that is the measure of right and wrong.

(Bentham, 1776)

And he wrote this about Dostoevsky:

In their zealous promotion of this greatest happiness, western social reformers – when calculating the greatest happiness of society – had treated the destinies of individuals as interchangeable units. The destinies and suffering of the few, the useless, the weak, the humble, and indeed the criminal … were implicitly disregarded. Dostoevsky's work could indeed be described as a continuous attempt to render plausible in all its implications a very simple idea: the harm done to the humblest and least significant human being can never in any circumstances be justified by any advantage derived from it by others.

(Katkov, 1951)

Here we begin to touch not only on medicine and healthcare, but also on the power of literature (Nussbaum, 1997). Healthcare professionals become very familiar with the destinies and suffering of the weak and the humble and the extent to which their subjective experience and their needs, hopes and fears are so often marginalised and neglected within a streamlined and industrialised healthcare system.

The great Polish poet Zbigniew Herbert endured the Soviet dictatorship and in 1974, he published a poem called *Damastes (also known as Procrustes) Speaks*. He describes inventing a bed with the measurements of a perfect man. He catches unwary travellers, and in order to make them fit his perfect bed, he has to stretch the limbs of some and cut the legs of others. Inevitably some of his 'patients' died – but the more that did so

the more I was certain my research was right
the goal was noble progress requires victims

By describing the victims as patients, he clearly identifies the brutal utopian reformer Procrustes as a doctor, which is profoundly disturbing.

The poem ends with the chilling prophecy that others will continue his work, and bring it to a 'successful' conclusion.

Sadly, even tragically, that is exactly what medicine seems to have gone on to do. The world of guidelines and targets and payment by results is in the process of bringing 'the task so wonderfully begun to its end'. It is, of course, essential to remain committed to the integrity and usefulness of medical science which has achieved enormous success through the application of general rules to individuals. Yet these undoubted achievements, as the poem suggests, have come at the price of annihilating and trivialising individual difference and the fundamental importance of the subjective experience of illness.

Too often, we seem content to dispense with any attempt to reach or acknowledge the subjective self of the person that we are attempting to diagnose and treat.

I fear that Popper's utopian engineering is alive and well within medicine and its hallmarks are a vision of the perfect human body and the perfect human life and a conviction that we know how other people should lead their lives. As doctors, we claim to know with frightening conviction and certainty what health is and how it is achieved.

The political theorist Herbert Marcuse was born into a Jewish family in Berlin in 1898. He moved into exile in the United States in 1934 when his academic position became untenable under the Third Reich. In his book *One Dimensional Man*, published in 1964, Marcuse described totalitarianism:

> 'Totalitarian' is not only a terroristic political coordination of society, but also a non-terroristic economic-technical coordination which operates through the manipulation of needs by vested interests.

This seems to me to be what large tracts of our healthcare systems have become: the vested financial interests of the medical industrial complex (Ehrenreich and Ehrenreich, 1971) drive the manipulation of need, the rules and the quality standards to which professionals are subjected, and the relentless widening of diagnostic categories that culminates in overdiagnosis and overtreatment. To give just one of many possible examples, back in 1999, Dartmouth researchers Lisa Schwarz and Steven Woloshin published a paper investigating the effects of changing disease definitions for four major conditions: diabetes, hypertension, hypercholesterolaemia and being overweight (Schwarz and Woloshin, 1999). The lowering of the thresholds for making a diagnosis created 32 million more patients just in the United States. And this was before the invention of pre-diabetes. By screening for risk, extending disease definitions, relabelling risk factors as diseases and applying disease labels to what were previously considered to be ordinary human experiences, we have allowed tests to displace listening, number to displace description, technology to displace touch, the objective to displace the subjective, and huge amounts of money to be made.

George Orwell's trenchant vision of a dystopic totalitarian future entitled *1984* was published on 8 June 1949. Ten days later, the American critic Lionel Trilling reviewed it for the *New Yorker* magazine. Trilling wrote:

> He is saying, indeed, something no less comprehensive than this: that Russia, with its idealistic social revolution now developed into a police state, is but the image of the impending future and that the ultimate threat to human freedom may well come from a similar and even more massive development of the social idealism of our democratic culture.
>
> (Trilling, 1949)

Arguably, the current ascendancy of ever more medical technology, which seeks to manipulate the human body as a machine rather than a self, is just such a manifestation of dangerous social idealism.

Trilling continued:

> The essential point of Nineteen Eighty-Four is just this, the danger of the ultimate and absolute power which the mind can develop when it frees itself from conditions, from the bondage of things and history.

The sorts of measurement which underpin the imperatives of contemporary medicine – blood pressure, serum cholesterol, bone density, PHQ9 depression score, body mass index, estimated glomerular filtration rate, just to mention a few, are all held to be universally applicable whatever the circumstance of the individual life to which they are applied. They are in Trilling's words 'freed from conditions' and therefore dangerous. People become reduced to numbers and Popper's actual living person disappears: the subjective self is missing.

Writing about the development and use of psychological tests, Tor-Johan Ekeland, Norwegian professor of psychology, describes such measurements as rendering:

> individuals into knowledge as objects of a hierarchical and normative gaze. The individuality is no longer unique and beyond knowledge, but can be known, mapped, calibrated, evaluated, quantified, predicted and managed. They become techniques for the disciplining of human difference.
>
> (Ekeland, 2004)

Biological variation and individuality has been appropriated to the causes of commercial profit and of lifestyle and political conformity. Physicians may not be driving this process but they are certainly colluding.

Abraham Verghese, Professor for the Theory and Practice of Medicine at Stanford, was born in Ethiopia of Indian parents but was forced to leave Ethiopia in 1974 during his third year at medical school because of the advent of the military government and extreme political instability. He, too, seems very aware of the extent to which the purging of the subjective self within contemporary healthcare systems becomes a tragedy not only for the sick but also for their doctors.

> People will say, 'He or she never listened to me.' 'He or she never laid a hand on me.' 'He or she had one foot in the door, one foot out of the door.' It is a failure of recognition of their being, and a failure of making use of our being, making use of our sense of self as physicians, as caregivers.
>
> (Verghese, 2016)

It seems more than a coincidence that so many writers who have been exposed to the perils of excessive political authoritarianism attach so much importance to the actual living person and his or her elusive selfhood. Modern bureaucratic societies 'privilege process, order and efficiency over morals, responsibility and care for the other' (Davis and Campbell, 2017) and so do modern bureaucratic healthcare systems and it is these priorities that drive the suppression of subjective experience and the risk of social totalitarianism.

So to summarise, the suppression of the self and of the importance of subjective experience within medicine suggests the development of a dangerous manifestation of social totalitarianism within contemporary healthcare. If these trends are to be resisted and mitigated, we will need to pay much more attention to the importance of intersubjective dialogue at every level of the health service.

Recovering the self

The American physician Eric Cassell describes the nature of suffering:

> We all recognize certain injuries that almost invariably cause suffering: the death or suffering of loved ones, powerlessness, helplessness, hopelessness, torture, the loss of a life's work, deep betrayal, physical agony, isolation, homelessness, memory failure, and unremitting fear. Each touches features common to us all, yet each contains features that must be defined in terms of a specific person at a specific time.
>
> (Cassell, 1991)

The attempt to relieve suffering is the moral core of clinical work yet suffering is almost completely absent from biomedical science and from the evidence-based guidelines which are derived from that science. The experience of suffering is bound to the self so that healthcare that minimises the importance of the self risks increasing rather than reducing suffering. In his essay about the Mexican artist Frida Kahlo, John Berger suggests that her painting expresses the human experience of pain, in all its various dimensions. Berger writes:

> the sharing of pain is one of the essential preconditions for a refinding of dignity and hope. Much pain is unshareable. But the will to share pain is shareable. And from that inevitably inadequate sharing comes a resistance.
>
> (Berger, 1998)

And it is 'the will to share pain' that both clinician and patient selves must bring to their meeting if suffering is to be located and, to at least some extent, relieved.

Most clinicians are not biomedical scientists: they have a different responsibility which is to attempt to relieve distress and suffering and, to this end, to enable the sick to benefit from advances in biomedical science while protecting people from its harms. Clinicians need to be able to see and hear each successive patient in the fullness of their humanity, to minimise fear, to locate hope (however limited), to explain symptoms and diagnoses in language that make sense to each different patient, to witness courage and endurance and to accompany suffering. There is no biomedical evidence that I know of that helps with any of this.

Philosopher Stephen Toulmin has warned about the need to:

> acknowledge and respect the essential differences between scientific and medical knowledge – notably, the physician's complex but indispensable fusion of the theoretical and the practical, the general and the particular, the universal and the existential.
>
> (Toulmin, 1993)

And he emphasises the importance of making it clear:

> just how far the fusion of medicine with biological science can afford to go, if it is not to destroy the essential character of medical practice and understanding.
>
> (Toulmin, 1993)

This was written more than 20 years ago but the warning does not seem to have been heard. The apparent determination to minimise the importance of the subjectivity of both patients and doctors has brought us to the point of teetering on the brink of this destruction.

Any hope of the necessary recovery of the self will rely on a commitment to deontology, to attention and to authentic dialogue.

Deontology

Health service policy in general and evidence-based medicine in particular are founded either on Benthamite utilitarian values of seeking to achieve the greatest benefit for the greatest number or on egalitarian values recognising equal rights to healthcare across society, and, in practice, most often on a rather confused mixture of the two. However, the task of the clinician is to engage with the detail of the fears, hopes, needs and values of each individual patient and, within any consultation, the moral obligation of the professional is to do his or her best for that particular real living person. Hence clinicians tend to adopt an ethical framework that is primarily deontological (Kelly *et al.*, 2015) with moral obligations that respond to the ethical commitment of the clinician to the individual patient. This is in line with the famous Second Formulation of Immanuel Kant's Categorical Imperative:

> Act in such a way that you always treat humanity, whether in your own person or in the person of any other, never simply as a means, but always at the same time as an end.
>
> (Kant, 1785)

The theologian Paul Tillich was born in Germany but when Hitler came to power in 1933, he was dismissed from his post as Professor of Theology at the University of Frankfurt and subsequently at the age of 47 moved his family to America. Tillich echoes Kant and describes:

> the unconditional imperative to acknowledge every person as a person. If we ask for the contents given by this absolute, we find, first, something negative – the command not to treat a person as a thing. This seems little, but it is much.
>
> (Tillich, 1969)

For healthcare professionals, if we are to find ways to resist the rules-based totalitarianism of contemporary healthcare, the imperative is that we treat our patients 'always at the same time as an end' whatever else we seek to achieve. And also that we treat ourselves, ourselves as doctors and other healthcare professionals, as an end and do not allow ourselves to be treated simply as a means. My contention is that contemporary healthcare systems have a destructive tendency to treat both patients and professionals as means to some other greater purpose, and neglect, at the same time, to treat them as ends in themselves. When we treat another person as an end in themselves, we embark on recovering the self and the subjectivity of both patients and doctors. Sadly, all this seems poorly understood and little appreciated by those policy-makers whose priorities are situated at the population or societal level. Yet, without this foundation in deontology, patients would find themselves unable to trust clinicians and the result would be, among much else, less efficiency at a societal level (Kushner, 1981).

Attention

If healthcare systems are to treat people as ends in themselves and thereby recover the self and respect the subjectivity of both patients and professionals, the primary requirement is that we should pay genuine attention to each other. The fine-grained particularity of each unique human self is emphasised in a 1959 children's book by the American absurdist writer Dr Seuss:

> There is no-one alive
> who is youer than you!
>
> (Seuss, 1959)

I mention this apparent triviality to assert the importance of the first and second person pronouns, *you* and *I*, which are the stuff of biography, of human relationships and of clinical medicine, rather than the impersonal third person of *he*, *she* or *it*, which is the stuff of biology and biomedical science. The only agent who can pay attention to a subject is another subject. There can be no room for the subjectivity of the patient unless there is room for the subjectivity of the doctor.

In his 1902 short story *Tomorrow* the great Polish/British novelist, Joseph Conrad, wrote:

Every mental state, even madness, has its equilibrium based upon self-esteem. Its disturbance causes unhappiness.

(Conrad, 1902)

I want to argue that this equilibrium, based on self-esteem, is vital to the health and well-being not only of patients but also of doctors. Esteem implies being valued and respected and, at least to some extent, as Conrad recognised, all human beings need a sense of themselves which includes at least some element of self-esteem. And this includes a sense of being worthy of the attention of others, as emphasised by the French philosopher Simone Weil in an essay written between 1942 and 1943:

'You do not interest me.' No man can say these words to another without committing a cruelty and offending against justice.

(Weil, 2003a)

In my professional life, I have been guilty of many such failures of attention, when preoccupied, working under pressure, feeling unwell myself, or otherwise distracted. The most striking example was my failure to pay appropriate attention to a patient who I will call Millie and who taught me a very important lesson.

My pivotal consultation with Millie occurred many years ago. She was very well-known to our practice team but, in fact, I knew very little about her. She was not actually registered with me but her own GP was away for three months on sabbatical leave and Millie had opted to see me in the interim. She was in her early seventies and I knew vaguely that her tyrannical mother had died relatively recently in her nineties. I also knew, even more vaguely, that Millie had had a prolonged admission to mental hospital in her early adult life for reasons that were far from clear. For the rest of her life she had lived with her mother until the latter's death. She now lived alone.

Millie made appointments to see me every week or two for no very clear reason and I was just trying to tide her over until her own doctor returned. Yet I was having the greatest difficulty in finishing the consultations in anything like the standard ten minutes. After a succession of these unsatisfactory meetings, she arrived one day, sat down and, to my shame, I immediately began to try and find a way of ending the consultation. At this point Millie did something remarkable and absolutely unprecedented in my experience. She got up from her chair, turned round and sat back down on my lap. There could not have been a clearer plea for attention.

After I had got over my initial astonishment, I suggested that Millie should go back to her own chair and that we should start again. Belatedly, I asked her a few simple questions about herself and her life. I learnt that she had one brother who had married and moved away, of whom she was fond but who she saw only very occasionally. And I learnt that she was then living two streets from where she had been born and that she had only been out of London once in her whole life, on a daytrip to Margate before the war. I was astonished for a second time in not much more than as many minutes. Combined with her by now obvious loneliness, this seemed the most profound geographical deprivation. I felt a surge of respect for her uncomplaining endurance. This fragment of recognition was all she needed. Our relationship was transformed and she no longer needed to come so often because I had finally glimpsed a tiny part of the reality of her life and made a small step towards recognising her as a very special self.

Before that transformative consultation, Millie would surely have recognised the predicament described by Isaiah Berlin:

> What I may seek to avoid is simply being ignored, or patronized, or despised, or being taken too much for granted – in short, not being treated as an individual, having my uniqueness insufficiently recognized, being classed as a member of some featureless amalgam, a statistical unit without identifiable, specifically human features and purposes of my own.
>
> (Berlin, 1969)

I will never forget Millie, nor that particular consultation, nor the lesson that she taught me: attention is essential and is profoundly rewarding to both patients and clinician.

Simone Weil described attention as 'moral concentration' and she elaborates on the challenge and the power of the degree of attention needed to recover the self:

> Those who are unhappy have no need for anything in this world but people capable of giving them their attention. The capacity to give one's attention to a sufferer is a very rare and difficult thing; it is almost a miracle; it is a miracle. Nearly all those who think they have this capacity do not possess it. Warmth of heart, impulsiveness, pity are not enough.
>
> (Weil, 2003b)

Weil would certainly have been less than impressed by my initial performance with Millie when I could not even summon up warmth of heart or pity, let alone genuine attention.

In *The Sovereignty of the Good*, British novelist and philosopher Iris Murdoch makes clear the extent to which we can regard attention as the antidote to the threat of totalitarianism:

> I have used the word 'attention', which I borrow from Simone Weil, to express the idea of a just and loving gaze directed upon an individual reality. I believe this to be the characteristic and proper mark of the active moral agent.
>
> (Murdoch, 1970)

And she goes on to describe the workings of attention:

> if we consider what the work of attention is like, how continuously it goes on, and how imperceptibly it builds up structures of value round about us, we shall not be surprised that at crucial moments of choice most of the business of choosing is already over.
>
> (Murdoch, 1970)

Arthur Kleinman, professor of both anthropology and cross-cultural psychiatry at Harvard, points out how difficult it is to sustain the required degree of attention when surrounded by the conflicting demands of a pressured healthcare system:

> the priorities of the practitioner lead to selective attention to the patient's account, so that some aspects are carefully listened for and heard (sometimes when they are not spoken), while other things that are said – and even repeated – are literally not heard.
>
> (Kleinman, 1988)

Such failures of attention to the subjective reality of the patient can have serious repercussions. As John Berger noted:

> Good general diagnosticians are rare, not because most doctors lack medical knowledge, but because most are incapable of taking in all the possibly relevant facts – emotional, historical, environmental as well as physical.
>
> (Berger and Mohr, 1967)

If these crucial dimensions of subjective experience are ignored, a key aetiological factor may be missed so that the diagnosis becomes partial or inadequate, or even wrong. While an ethical framework of deontology and a receptive attitude of moral concentration help to create John Berger's intersubjective 'will to share', the actual work of recovering the self, depends on dialogue because, at its most basic, it is my response to your words that tells you whether I am paying attention to you or not. And vice versa.

Dialogue

Looking at the several ontologies of the self which Christopher Dowrick presents in a later chapter, I find the notion of the social/distributed self to be the most useful when facing the task of recovering the self within the daily realities of clinical practice. My pragmatic understanding is that the self is created within each human individual through interaction with the world and within human relationships. Babies become conscious of their place in the world through dialogue with the behaviours and responses of those around them. A brain is confined to each individual but I find it very helpful to think of mind as relational and oriented towards the world and others. The self-perception and self-esteem of those who are raised in a context of violence and abuse is likely to be very different from those lucky enough to grow up within a context of love, affection and positive regard. Throughout a life story, consciousness and memory combine to create a self with a remembered past and an imagined future.

> People came to presume that when they talked of their 'memories,' they meant experiences and learning that were carefully stored away in their brains and could be brought into consciousness, or made conscious. But this was to ignore the possibility that memories were in fact part of the very structure of consciousness: not only can there be no such thing as a memory without there being consciousness, but consciousness and memory are in a certain sense inseparable, and understanding one requires understanding the other....
>
> It is not that my memories exist as stored images in my brain, conscious or unconscious; the act of memory is one of my relating to myself, or to others, or to past experiences, or to previously perceived stimuli. This is the very essence of memory: its self-referential base, its self-consciousness, ever evolving and ever changing, intrinsically dynamic and subjective.
>
> (Rosenfield, 1992)

The dialogue between consciousness and memory is continuous and like all authentic dialogue reflects John Berger's description of drawing as 'a constant correcting of errors' (Berger, 2011). Our attempts to understand the world and those around us are subject to this 'constant correcting of errors', shifting and adjusting to the unfolding of events and relationships. Yet, trauma of any sort has the potential to wound not only the body but also the self, distorting both memory and consciousness. Language is acquired through dialogue with others: within social networks that can be thought of as shared minds (Epstein, 2013). Perhaps these shared minds can also help in mending the distortions of a trauma-tised consciousness, as the correcting of errors becomes a social rather than a solitary activity.

Another patient taught me of the persistence of self-consciousness and memory even in extreme dementia. I will call her Laura.

Laura developed a severe dementing illness in her late seventies. Fortunately, she lived next door to her daughter and so was able to remain at home throughout her lengthy illness. Her dementia became so severe that she began to lose language and, at the point when only single words remained, one of her young lay carers had the wonderful idea of writing down every recognisable word that Laura said. The result was almost a poem made up of the names of her mother and sisters still remembered from her childhood, interspersed with words of affection which included darling and love. It was extraordinarily comforting as it seemed to imply that Laura's subjective experience was of love rather than distress.

We need at this point to go back to the beginnings of illness and the role of dialogue. Illness begins with the moment when subjective feelings are first articulated into thoughts of illness and thereby privately acknowledged as symptoms. Sensation hardens into a symptom, fear crystallises and becomes explicit. The interweaving of past, present and future, in memory and imagination, has a powerful effect on the manner and speed with which feelings become thoughts and perceptions become symptoms. What happened when I felt this sensation before? Did I feel foolish or relieved when it resolved – or both? Do the feelings seem similar to those described by my mother or father at the beginning of a serious illness? Has my closest friend been given a life-threatening diagnosis in recent months? Am I looking forward to some particularly important occasion which could be threatened by this new feeling? The dialogue at this point is all internal.

Each different self, aided and abetted by a variable combination of sensibility, preoccupation, fear, denial and stoicism, sets the boundary between the significant and the insignificant at a different point. Each of us allows a feeling to become a symptom at a different threshold.

Sooner or later, thoughts must become words in order to be shared within an external, interpersonal dialogue. What happens, what are the processes by which feelings become thoughts and thoughts become words? Each stage seems to require compression and reduction as the experiential is constrained within the linguistic. Thought lags behind feeling and words behind thought. The self attenuates: how much is lost and to what extent, if at all, is it possible to recover what is lost?

Subjective experience and the feelings it invokes are free-floating and infinite yet completely unique to the individual; concretised into thoughts, feelings begin to be both structured and restricted. The next step by which thoughts are further concretised into language imposes another layer of structure and restriction. Experience, feelings and thoughts are necessarily lonely and only when expressed in language can they be shared. Precisely because they are shared, words aspire to what is universal in human experience.

The Russian philosopher and semiotician, Mikhail Bakhtin (whom we have already met in Deborah Swinglehurst's chapter) analyses the dialogic nature of language. He describes the way in which words are changed and refracted by each usage – continually subject to both centripetal and centrifugal forces. As each one of us appropriates words for our own purposes, we add our own particular shade of meaning producing a centrifugal force which continually develops and fragments language; yet at the same time, all language is social and built on the attempt to achieve shared and centripetal understanding. Our subjective experience is necessarily lonely. Language – thoughts and feelings given substance as words – is our defence against that loneliness. Language is essential to the human struggle to feel less alone but also dependent on Berger's 'will to share'.

> The authentic environment of an utterance, the environment in which it lives and takes shape, is dialogized heteroglossia, anonymous and social as

language, but simultaneously concrete, filled with specific content and accented as an individual utterance.

(Bakhtin, 1981)

The words spoken by those who are sick are the closest we can come to the human experience of illness. They represent only a shadow of the totality of that experience, but they express the most that we are able, through language, to share.

Once articulated, the power of words to make us feel less alone is astonishing and consoling. They are both the means and the ends of the human compulsion to search for meaning. They form the map which outlines our understanding and, at the same time, guides our search for more. Words help us to make sense of our daily experience of joy and suffering and make it absolutely clear that those experiences are shared, at least partially, and that, to this extent, we are less alone.

However, as soon as thoughts are expressed as words, they become public and there is the possibility of embarrassment and of appearing foolish. Symptoms are driven by fear, but if the fear turns out to be groundless, one may feel foolish. Intimate relationships enable embarrassment to be risked in a way that public relationships do not, which is why the relationship between doctor and patient, although formal, must remain intimate. And because it takes time to develop the trust that is essential to intimacy, continuity of care (Starfield, 2011) remains fundamentally important.

> Men and women ... have words. With their words they change everything, and nothing. Whatever the circumstances, words add and take away. Either spoken words or ones heard in the head. They are always incongruous, because they never fit. This is why words cause pain and why they offer salvation.
>
> (Berger, 1990)

And expressing the same contradiction:

> Words can cause trouble like large rocks in one's path.
> Wrong: Words can clear the largest rocks out of the way.
> Wrong again: Words can turn into dark chasms unbridgeable for a whole lifetime.
> We know very little about the power and the destructiveness of words.
>
> (Vesaas, 1971)

Meaning is inevitably changed during the movement of dialogue from private to public, from inner to outer, and from Epstein's whole mind to shared mind (Epstein, 2013). The challenge for the listener is to minimise that change and to approach as close as possible to the inner, private experience. And having listened, the next daunting challenge is to find words to contain what we have heard and to demonstrate and communicate our understanding. The finding of words is always a subjective activity. Listening, testing and then correcting understanding is a continuous dialogical process and, as philosopher and patient Kay Toombs points out, dialogue is completely different from the all too common clinical interrogation:

> it is important to note the difference between interrogation and dialogue. Questions which admit of only 'yes' or 'no' answers do not allow the respondent to provide a description of his or her experience.... If the physician is to learn something about the patient's experience he or she must initiate a dialogue with the patient – a dialogue that allows the patient to provide a first person narrative of the illness.
>
> (Toombs, 1993)

Dialogue allows the patient to reveal the experience of the subjective self, but the extent and nature of any dialogue is affected by language, culture and context. Clinicians need to try always to:

> notice the subtle ways in which language orders perceptions and how language constructs social interaction. Symptoms are situated in culture and context, and trends in modern everyday life modify symptom understanding continuously ... a symptom can only be understood by attention to the social context in which the symptom emerges and the dialogue through which it is negotiated.
>
> (Malterud *et al.*, 2015)

Within every clinical consultation both professional and patient oscillate between perceiving the human body as an object and as a subject. When the body is perceived as an object, the gaze of biomedical science sees only what the particular patient has in common with other patients. On the other hand, when we seek to understand the body as a subject, we speak about what is unique about this person – their life context, its story and the meanings that adhere to both. The perspective is dialogical and intersubjective involving two unique subjects – the patient – and the professional.

Each subject brings their own history and experience to the dialogue. Australian novelist David Malouf describes the way in which:

> Even the least event had lines, all tangled, going back into the past, and beyond that into the unknown past, and other lines leading out, also tangled, into the future. Every moment was dense with causes, possibilities, consequences; too many, even in the simplest case, to grasp.
>
> (Malouf, 1990)

Within the dialogue between a patient and a doctor, two sets of lines tangle. All too often, we, as doctors, can only make sense of what is happening to the patient if we can follow at least a few of these tangled lines – if we can follow the story over time – and if we remain always aware of the effects of our own particular tangled lines.

> Irene was my patient for more than 25 years until her death in October 2001. She had been subjected to the predations of interpersonal and structural violence since childhood – and the multiple adverse experiences of her childhood played out through her biology and culminated in her early death in her 50s. She and I were on the local maternity ward together 40 years ago. In 1977, I was having my first child, she her third and last – both were girls. Sadly her child was born with severe learning disability. After Irene died, her husband gave me a copy of their wedding photo. They had met when their children from their previous relationships were in the care of the local authority. She is smoking in her wedding photo and this suggests both the trauma of her abusive childhood and the nature of her terminal illness.

Yet, none of this tells us anything about Irene's enormous reserves of courage that I slowly learned to appreciate over 25 years of intersubjective dialogue. I also learned to understand that her fears when she was dying had nothing to do with the imminence of death, but to do with the care of her youngest child and whether her husband would be able to cope with the burden of responsibility that she had shouldered without complaint for more than 20 years.

To care for Irene adequately, I had to appreciate her both as a bodily object beset by various illnesses and diseases which included bronchiectasis, hypertension and lung and mouth cancer; but also, as a particular human subject with a particular life story and extraordinary resources of courage and endurance.

Sadly, as Stefan Hjørleifsson, Kjersti Lea and David Misselbrook discuss elsewhere in this book, medicine and medical science have had a strong bias towards approaching the body as an object and has tended to marginalise the importance the subjective perspective. The result is the missing self that we are trying to recover. Both perspectives are essential to effective care but the oscillation is essential because each gaze corrects the other. The same is true of the use of words in the consultation.

Norwegian general practitioner John Nessa has written about talk as medical work and he insists that:

> Clinical medicine is talk and gaze as an integrated whole.
>
> (Nessa, 1999)

He also notes that dialogue is only genuine when both parties are open to be changed by it, when there is the 'will to share':

> a dialogue is an interpersonal mode of being which at its best may be called authentic interaction. The 'magic' of authentic interaction is that we do not

completely control it as individuals, but are caught up in it and give in to its own movement.

(Nessa and Malterud, 1998)

It seems important to understand that this description of 'authentic interaction' is completely incompatible with the sort of didactic consultation that aims to achieve compliance with a guideline, a target or a treatment plan.

Each patient self has fears, hopes, preferences and values and so does each doctor self. If treatment is to be appropriate, the dialogue between patient and doctor should include a willingness to share these subjective attributes and a willingness to negotiate differences. If the priorities of either party remain hidden or are simply assumed the subsequent decisions risk being dangerously misguided, as when:

> one medical value – longevity – has implicitly dominated the discussion of the proper treatment of many diseases, including breast cancer, and obliterated the consideration of all other values.

(Katz, 1984, p. 96)

The more we understand about the extent to which individual biography affects biology, the more important understanding subjective experience and recovering the self becomes to effective medical care. The irony is that the profligate destruction of the traditions of relationship-based intersubjective healthcare is occurring just as science itself is beginning to explain the mechanism of those aspects of medical practice which have come to be regarded as unscientific and therefore redundant.

As psychoneuroimmunology gradually unpicks the extraordinarily intricate interactions between the immune system, the autonomic nervous system and the subjective experience of the individual, the more we can understand the power of both positive and negative psychological states to promote or undermine the healthy functioning of the human body (Ulvestad, 2012). It becomes increasingly clear that physical and psychological stressors act on the body through the same pathways and that the customary distinction between the physical and the psychological is both illusory and meaningless. Supportive personal intersubjective relationships, sustained by authentic dialogue, and including, one must presume, relationships between doctors and patients, diminish negative emotions and promote health through a positive impact on immune function. And interestingly, dialogue with the natural world can have a similar beneficial effect as evidenced by research showing that access to green spaces appears to reduce the damaging health effects caused by socioeconomic inequality (Mitchell and Popham, 2008).

Allostasis is the process by which physiological functions respond to challenge and it seems to be mediated by multiple neurological, hormonal and immune mechanisms, but the body's capacity for allostasis is limited and can be overloaded by continuous and excessive stress. Biographical stress has many causes including grief, loss, structural violence and interpersonal conflict, and its effect on biology seems to be mediated by allostatic overload (McEwen, 1998). A recent paper from Norway examined the effect of 'existential unease' on the development of multimorbidity. The concept of existential unease was used to capture lack of self-esteem, well-being, meaning and/or social interrelatedness. The findings supported the researchers' initial hypothesis that existential unease contributes to allostatic load and thereby increases the susceptibility to disease across a life-course:

> From the perspective of primary care, our findings highlight the importance of an encompassing, person-centred approach, not the least in the face of complex disease and multimorbidity. Subjective experiences pertaining to the self, one's life project and relationships with other people apparently matter, in a literal sense. As we conclude so, it is, however, not our intention to medicalise every aspect of the human lifeworld and suggest that human happiness should be subjected to systematic, medical surveillance. What we hope to contribute to is a more comprehensive medical understanding that does justice to the human nature. This is ultimately a fundamental prerequisite for good healthcare.
>
> (Tomasdottir *et al.*, 2016)

Clinicians need to understand the subjective experience of the patient's self in order to recognise sources of biographical stress in the hope of being able, at least to some extent, to modify or mitigate them.

Conclusion

To conclude, let us return to Joseph Conrad's emphasis on the importance of self-esteem. When the self-esteem of patients is undermined by cruelty, violence, injustice, stigma or shame, well-being and health can be rapidly undermined. The most vulnerable patients presenting as patients in general practice have had very little sense of being valued and respected in their lives and, perhaps, one of the most powerful interventions the doctor can offer is communicating a genuine positive regard imbued with esteem. Similarly, in the wake of the increasing marketisation and bureaucratisation of healthcare, doctors have been portrayed as less and less worthy of esteem with any sense of the importance of their subjectivity being minimised in the interests of efficiency. The illusion is that any doctor will do and self-esteem on the part of doctors has been portrayed as arrogance and paternalism. Yet, without it, doctors become demoralised and unhappy and less able to engage their patients in a genuinely intersubjective therapeutic dialogue.

Both health and ill-health are socially constructed within relationships including those created within clinical consultations. The subjective experience of both patients and doctors matters. Each needs to recognise the other and to feel recognised.

Note

Some material in this chapter was first presented in a keynote lecture to the 2016 International Conference on Communication in Healthcare in Heidelberg, Germany. The text of the lecture has been published in the journal *Patient Education and Counselling* (Heath, 2017).

Key learning points

- Totalitarianism is leading to the obliteration of the doctor and patient self within contemporary healthcare:
  - Healthcare is increasingly subsumed within commercial vested interests.
  - We can learn from writers who have escaped from totalitarian systems.
  - Pragmatic changes to social and health care are safer than utopian social reform programmes.

- To recover the self we need to:
  - recognise the nature of suffering
  - acknowledge the difference between scientific and medical knowledge
  - operate within an ethical framework based on moral obligations to patients
  - pay genuine attention to each other
  - understand how dialogue is essential in generating meaning
  - be aware of how biographical stress influences our sense of self
  - recognise that the self-esteem of both doctors and patients is essential to intersubjective therapeutic dialogue.

References

Bakhtin, M.M. 1981. *The dialogic imagination: four essays.* Austin: University of Texas Press.

Bauman, Z. 2011. Capitalism has learned to create host organisms. *Guardian* [online]. Available at: www.theguardian.com/commentisfree/2011/oct/18/capitalism-parasite-hosts (accessed 12 January 2017).

Bentham, J. 1776. *A fragment on government.* London: T. Payne.

Berger, J. 1990. *Lilac and flag.* New York: Pantheon Books.

Berger, J. 1998. Frida Kahlo, in *The shape of a pocket.* London: Bloomsbury, 2002: 157–64.

Berger, J. 2011. *Newsnight*, 2011. [TV programme] BBC, 27 May. Available at: www.youtube.com/watch?v=U7LZxCUApds (accessed 19 January 2017).

Berger, J. and Mohr, J. 1967. *A fortunate man.* Harmondsworth: Penguin.

Berlin, I. 1969. Two concepts of liberty. *In: Four essays on liberty.* Oxford: Oxford University Press.

Cassell, E. 1991. *The nature of suffering.* New York: Oxford University Press.

Conrad, J. 1902. Tomorrow. *Pall Mall Magazine* [online]. Available at: https://ebooks.adelaide.edu.au/c/conrad/joseph/c75tm/ (accessed 12 January 2017).

Davis, M. and Campbell, T. 2017. Zygmunt Bauman obituary. *Guardian*, 16 January 2017. Available at: www.theguardian.com/education/2017/jan/15/zygmunt-bauman-obituary?CMP=share_btn_tw (accessed 16 January 2017).

Ehrenreich, B. and Ehrenreich, J. 1971. *The American health empire*. New York: Vintage Books.

Ekeland, T.-J. 2004. *Epistemological errors and the return of the Jedi. Problems in mainstream psychology and implications for practice.* Keynote speech at Bergen Symposium on Cultural and Critical Psychology. Exploring Psychological Perspectives and Their Practical Consequences, University of Bergen, 1–2 June 2004.

Eliot, T.S. 1945. *What is a classic? An address delivered before the Virgil Society on the 16th of October 1944.* London: Faber & Faber.

Epstein, R.M. 2013. Whole mind and shared mind in clinical decision-making. *Patient Education and Counselling*, 90 (2): 200–6.

Heath, I. 2017. The missing person: The outcome of the rule-based totalitarianism of too much contemporary healthcare. *Patient Education and Counselling*, 3 April. [Epub ahead of print].

Holmes, J. 2014. *The therapeutic imagination*. Hove: Routledge.

Kant, I. 1785. *Groundwork of the metaphysic of morals.*

Katkov, G. 1951. The Spiritual Message of Dostoevsky. *The Listener*, 1059–60.

Katz, J. 1984. *The silent world of doctor and patient*. New York: The Free Press.

Kelly, M., Heath, I., Howick, J. and Greenhalgh, T. 2015. The importance of values in evidence-based medicine. *BMC Medical Ethics*, 16 (1). Available at: www.ncbi.nlm.nih.gov/pmc/articles/PMC4603687/

Kleinman, A. 1988. *The illness narratives*. New York: Basic Books.

Kushner, T. 1981. Doctor-patient relationships in general practice–a different model. *Journal of Medical Ethics*, 7 (3): 128–31.

Malouf, D. 1990. *The great world*. London: Chatto & Windus.

Malterud, K., Guassora, A., Graungaard, A. and Reventlow, S. 2015. Understanding medical symptoms: a conceptual review and analysis. *Theoretical Medicine and Bioethics*, 36 (6): 411–24.

Marcuse, H. 1964. *One-dimensional man*. London: Routledge & Kegan Paul.

McEwen, B. 1998. Protective and Damaging Effects of Stress Mediators. *New England Journal of Medicine*, 338 (3): 171–9.

McGregor, S. 2001. Neoliberalism and healthcare. *International Journal of Consumer Studies*, 25: 82–9.

McKee, M. and Clarke, A. 1995. Guidelines, enthusiasms, uncertainty, and the limits to purchasing. *BMJ*, 310 (6972): 101–4.

Mitchell, R. And Popham, F. 2008. Effect of exposure to natural environment on health inequalities: an observational population study. *The Lancet*, 372 (9650): 1655–60.

Morris, D.B. 1998. *Illness and culture in the postmodern age*. Berkeley: University of California Press.

Murdoch, I. 1970. *The sovereignty of the good*. London: Routledge & Kegan Paul.

Nessa, J. 1999. *Talk as medical work*. Bergen: University of Bergen.

Nessa, J. and Malterud, K. 1998. Tell me what's wrong with me: a discourse analysis approach to the concept of patient autonomy. *Journal of Medical Ethics*, 24 (6): 394–400.

Nussbaum, M. 1986. *The Fragility Of Goodness*. Cambridge: Cambridge University Press.

Nussbaum, M. 1997. *Poetic justice: the literary imagination and public life*. Boston: Beacon Press.

Popper, K. 1945. *The open society and its enemies.* London: Routledge.

Rosenfield, I. 1992. *The strange, familiar, and forgotten: an anatomy of consciousness.* New York: Knopf.

Santayana, G. 1980. *Reason in common sense.* New York: Dover Publications.

Schwartz, L.M. and Woloshin, S. 1999. Changing disease definitions: implications for disease prevalence. Analysis of the Third National Health and Nutrition Examination Survey, 1988–1994. *Effective Clinical Practice,* 2 (2): 76–85.

Seuss, Dr. 1959. *Happy birthday to you!* New York: Random House.

Starfield, B. 2011. Is Patient-Centered Care the Same As Person-Focused Care? *The Permanente Journal,* 15 (2): 63–9.

Steiner, G. 1967. *Language and silence: essays 1958–1966.* London: Faber & Faber.

Tillich, P. 1969. *My search for absolutes.* New York: Simon and Schuster.

Tomasdottir, M., Sigurdsson, J., Petursson, H., Kirkengen, A., Ivar Lund Nilsen, T., Hetlevik, I. and Getz, L. 2016. Does 'existential unease' predict adult multimorbidity? Analytical cohort study on embodiment based on the Norwegian HUNT population. *BMJ Open,* 6 (11): p.e012602.

Toombs, S.K. 1993. *The meaning of illness.* Dordrecht: Kluwer Academic.

Toulmin, S. 1993. Knowledge and art in the practice of medicine: clinical judgment and historical reconstruction. *In*: Delkeskamp-Hayes C. and Gardell Cutter M.A. (eds). *Science, technology, and the art of medicine.* Dordrecht: Kluwer Academic Publishers.

Trilling, L. 1949. Orwell on the future. Review of Nineteen Eighty-Four, by George Orwell. *New Yorker* 25 (June 18, 1949), 78: 81–3.

Ulvestad, E. 2012. Psychoneuroimmunology: the experiential dimension. *Methods Mol Biol,* 934: 21–37.

Verghese, A. 2016. I Carry Your Heart. *JAMA Cardiology,* 1 (2): 213.

Vesaas, T. 1971. *The boat in the evening.* London: Peter Owen Publishers.

Weil, S. 2003a, written 1942–3. Human Personality. *In*: Miles, S. (ed.) *Simone Weil: an anthology.* London: Penguin.

Weil, S. 2003b, written 1942. Reflections on the right use of school studies. *In*: Miles, S. (ed.) *Simone Weil: an anthology.* London: Penguin.

5　In defence of the conscious mind

David Misselbrook

Introduction

A young adult consults me – let's call him James. James is unhappy. His girlfriend died in a road accident and now, several weeks on, James feels low with early morning waking and some thoughts of self harm. He cannot concentrate, and his performance at his neuroscience degree course has declined. He has never felt like this before. He has been thinking about his problems and tells me 'I just can't snap out of it'. He does a PHQ-9 questionnaire for me and scores 16, indicating that he is moderately depressed. He himself has decided that his neurotransmitters are out of balance and wants to discuss starting a course of SSRIs (a class of modern, fairly safe, antidepressant).

Then I see Edith Brown. She has already consulted other doctors in this book. She is a 71-year-old widow who lives alone. She comes to see me for a medication review. She has multiple pathology including three previous TIAs. She has a long list of prescribed medications (Warfarin, Ramipril, Simvastatin, Atenolol, Amlodipine, Paracetamol, Codeine, Citalopram, Senna and Macrogol). Her neighbour pops in a couple of times a week. Her daughter, Emma, who lives 30 miles away, visits every weekend. Mrs Brown enjoys spending time with her grandchildren and volunteers in a local charity shop. But her medication causes postural dizziness and she finds it all a bit confusing. She is considering giving up her voluntary work as she fears she might fall or feel unwell in the shop.

My next patient, Mrs Sayyid, is in her late 80s. She is brought in by her daughter, Amal, who is finding it increasingly difficult to support her mother. Her mother's mild dementia is becoming worse. She repeats the same questions over and over again as she cannot remember the answer. She is distressed that her husband (who has been dead for many years) has 'gone missing'. Amal says, 'She isn't herself anymore doctor. It is as if she is the one who is missing.'

As we practice medicine most of us don't want to get bogged down by theory – we just want to get on and do our best for our patients. We'll use whatever maps seem best. We are grateful for the sparkling new maps provided by science that have transformed so much of our job. But sometimes the maps seem not to fit. Science is great for explaining how ACE inhibition strengthens a weakened myocardium, but it tells me little about how to mend a bereaved patient's broken heart. So should biomedicine be the sole basis for deciding my first two patients' needs? And I remain puzzled as how to answer Amal's uncertainty about her mother's changed identity.

Medicine, especially primary care medicine, is about people. Every day we see patients like James and Mrs. Brown and Mrs. Sayyid who we believe matter, because *people* matter. But sometimes biomedicine doesn't do people very well. And patients make choices that sometimes we disagree with but we still believe them to have dignity, always worthy of our respect and care.

But what if we are making a mistake? What if we humans are really just machines or ordinary animals, with nothing special about our humanity? What if our job is really no different from that of a car mechanic, or perhaps a vet? Is there anything special about being human? (Misselbrook, 2016, p. 39) This central issue relates to the nature of human consciousness. But, in the twenty-first century, this is a matter for disagreement and confusion.

There is a reason for this confusion. It is about what is real and how we can know things. Much of this chapter is about how scientific knowledge relates to other ways of knowing about the world. And answering the more fundamental question – *can* there be ways of knowing about the world other than science? We have to sort out a bit of theory before we can make sense of things.

The focus of this chapter is on the nature of human consciousness. Our problem is that our experience of our own human consciousness does not fit well with what we know through science. Including neuroscience (actually, *especially* neuroscience). Surely this is a problem? The philosopher David Chalmers has called this the 'hard problem of consciousness' (Chalmers, 1995). To be a good physicist you don't really need to think much about the nature of consciousness. Just do the science. But good doctors should pay some attention to this or they may find themselves tripped up by trying to use exclusively biomedical models that don't fit the needs of real people.

So this chapter examines a number of questions. How can we construct knowledge? What are the possible conceptual models for the nature of human consciousness? Can neuroscience give a complete account of consciousness? Does science have a privileged view of the world and could it be our only source of knowledge? If a pure neuroscience model of consciousness is inadequate, then what?

Strong consciousness

Throughout this chapter I will be referring to both 'mind' and 'consciousness'. The 'mind' to which I refer is our conscious mind – our self-aware mind. In referring to 'mind' I am referring to this property of self-aware consciousness, not primarily to the psychological or neurological mechanisms on which this consciousness depends. But why should doctors care about the nature of the conscious mind? Isn't it enough that we all inhabit our own minds? Cannot we just appeal to Descartes' 'I think, therefore I am' and leave it at that?

Unfortunately doctors do need some commitment to who the 'I' is in Descartes' saying. The debate about the nature of consciousness cannot be separated from the issue of the self – the focus of this book. Is my mind really the sort of thing that I instinctively experience it to be? Does the possession of human consciousness give me some degree of freedom, moral responsibility, human dignity? Or might these instinctive and obvious beliefs about my own nature actually be an error, just like humankind's obvious and common sense historical 'knowledge' that the sun circles the earth because we see it rise every morning?

The type of consciousness that I am defending I am calling 'strong consciousness'. By this I mean the presence of a mind that is a real thing in itself, capable not only of self-awareness but also some degree of freedom and choice, and thus moral responsibility, in a way than cannot be reduced only to deterministic biological functions of the brain. (By a determinist view I mean the theory that, whatever consciousness may be, it depends upon the function of a brain, a bodily organ made of physical matter that can *only* follow physical laws.) Determinists would say that the decisions that we think we make freely with our minds must actually be determined by predictable physical processes in the brain. So by this account my freedom is an illusion.

So if we disagree with determinism we must think that strong consciousness implies that there is more to my whole self than my physical body. Personhood (in a full sense), autonomy and responsibility are meaningless unless our consciousness is real in its own right and confers some degree of freedom, making us moral agents who therefore possess moral responsibility. But is this true, or should we just accept a deterministic view of the mind?

Doctors have both a practical and a moral need to take personhood seriously. We therefore need to understand the debate about the nature of human consciousness. In this chapter I claim that we need a commitment to a strong model of consciousness that sees human consciousness itself as an agent within the world. Such a view forms the conceptual basis for a proper account of personhood and thus for a richer notion of the proper tasks of medicine.

Consciousness as a problem to be solved: a modernistic view

Are matter and energy existing within space and time the only things that really exist? Analysis within a matter-energy within space-time model has been hugely successful in cosmology and physics. With our current models of star formation within the enormous number of galaxies emerging from the big bang we have developed a huge, rich and amazing cosmology that we have good reasons to believe is approximately true (though certainly not complete). Relativity enables us to understand space-time in a fuller way than our forebears. And quantum theory peels several further layers off the onion of small things, travelling towards a more fundamental understanding of the nature of matter-energy. The physical sciences work! But does a description of matter-energy existing within space-time give a *complete* account of the universe (i.e. leaving nothing out)? This view is called 'physicalism', and is one of this chapter's key concepts. I will support and expand on the critique of physicalism by Stefan Hjørleifsson and Kjersti Lea, presented in an earlier chapter of this book.

Most of science deals with matter-energy within space-time, so physicalism often seems to fit. This gives us an excellent basis for biomedicine in its project of describing bodily organs (including the brain) and their pathology. But as humans we realise that this does not give us a good basis for understanding that most vital aspect of our mind – our own self-awareness.

Medics have a tendency to privilege the biomedical elements of the bio-psycho-social model to which we pay lip service. In part this is due to our medical commitment to science as the 'best way of knowing' (Opel *et al.*, 2011). Yet much of the GP's work is best done using models from the humanities, the 'social sciences', or just our own humanity, none of which have the same foundation in the physical sciences. Therefore we are prone, perhaps unthinkingly, to see biomedical knowledge as 'hard' knowledge and the rest as 'soft' knowledge which is somehow not quite as respectable and must be given a lower seat at the table. My goal is to examine such thinking and explain why it is wrong.

We not only have mental processes but we realise that we are *aware* of our own mental processes. As Thomas Nagel (1974) puts it 'there is something that it is like' in being a particular person. This leaves a purely biological account of humanity with a problem, as it suggests the possibility that the mind cannot be seen as *nothing but* the physical organ of the brain. Let us examine this problem.

Thinking about thinking

Descartes (1596–1650) famously proposed that the mind was made of different stuff than the body – that the mind and the body were different substances (Descartes, 1641, Meditation 6). He saw our bodies as made of matter (*res extensa* or 'physical stuff') and our minds as made of something different that is not matter (*res cogitans* or 'thinking stuff'). This view is called 'dualism' – mind is different stuff from matter. So for Descartes matter must follow predictable physical laws but the mind has a different nature which enables it to be self-aware and to make free choices. Within 'me' as a totality there is an 'I myself', a mind aware of myself, free to choose how the 'bodily me' will act. For Descartes the thinking stuff *controlled* the physical stuff, thus the two were separate but interacting substances. This is called interactionism. This had an important influence on subsequent thought. Interactionism in one form or another is still our common sense way of thinking about the problem of minds that live with bodies.

In *A Treatise of Human Nature*, David Hume (1739) saw us as creatures of instinct and habit. He claimed that our beliefs are primarily the product of association and custom, and that our actions are determined by instinct, habit and emotion rather than by reason. Hume downgraded a sense of coherent and continuing personal identity or self. Hume argued that we construct such an identity for ourselves from the fleeting and unrelated series of perceptions contained in the mind.

In the nineteenth century Thomas Huxley (1874) suggested that our thoughts and feelings are simply the idle side effects of our actions and our brain states. He compared them to the whistle on the steam train: the whistle is a loud but irrelevant by product of the action of the train. Perhaps consciousness attracts our attention but doesn't drive the train? By this account our consciousness is not the thing we naturally take it to be, but it is a mere 'epiphenomenon' of the deterministic actions of our brain. An epiphenomenon is a secondary effect, a by-product, not having any real significance in itself. It wouldn't really matter whether the epiphenomenon was there or not – it plays no part in the real event (e.g. a rainbow is an epiphenomenon of rain, but it has no effect on the rain itself). So are we just 'conscious automata'? One could call this model of consciousness as an epiphenomenon 'mere consciousness', in distinction to my earlier description of 'strong consciousness'.

Gilbert Ryle

Perhaps the most important philosophical determinist of the 20th century was the Oxford philosopher Gilbert Ryle. His book (Ryle, 1949) *The Concept of Mind* was published in 1949, and has influenced philosophers and neuroscientists ever since.

Ryle argues that

> the physical world is a deterministic system, so the mental world must be a deterministic system. Bodies cannot help the modifications that they undergo, so minds cannot help pursing the careers fixed for them. *Responsibility, choice, merit* and *demerit* are therefore inapplicable concepts.
>
> (1949, Chapter I, 3 [Ryle's italics])

Ryle describes will or volition as 'an absurd hypothesis'. He famously describes Descartes concept of mind – interactionism via a *res cogitans* – as 'the ghost in the machine'. He regards this model as arising from a category error that wrongly insists that 'minds are not bits of clockwork, they are just bits of non-clockwork'.

To Ryle then, the idea of an autonomous self, based on a strong theory of consciousness, is laughable. The self is simply a term of convenience denoting our awareness of a deterministic process that bridges the brain's input and output. But this awareness is that of an observer, not an agent. My conscious self can be no freer to make choices than an apple is free to choose whether to stay on the branch or to fall. Some may stay and some may fall, but the laws of physics, chemistry and biology are entirely adequate to explain why.

Contemporary deterministic neuroscience

Neuroscience studies the workings of the brain using the techniques of the biological sciences. Our knowledge of the biology of the brain is increasing at an explosive pace. Neuroscience is busy translating the arguments of Ryle from the language of philosophy into the language of biology. It has advanced recently by techniques such as PET (Positron Emission Tomography) scanning, which show the activity, rather than just the structure, of the complex neural networks in the brain. Various groups of neuroscientists, psychologists and philosophers in the twentieth century seemed to be converging, from their different disciplines, towards a common position of brain determinacy and consciousness as epiphenomenalism (the view that consciousness is merely an epiphenomenon).

This view gained support from a remarkable experiment by Benjamin Libet, recently revisited by Patrick Haggard (Haggard *et al.*, 1999). Haggard was able to show that the brain commences the series of mental processes leading to a co-ordinated 'voluntary' action *before* the person themselves made the conscious decision to act. This supports the view that the brain is a complex but deterministic biological machine which generates consciousness, and with it a *spurious* sense of volition, as a by-product of its activities. Another example would be of 'blindsight' – the label for neurological damage where a person may have no visual data presented to his consciousness and yet be able to act on the basis of visual data that is clearly accessible to non-conscious brain pathways (Weiskrantz, 1990). As Daniel Dennett (1991), a pupil of Ryle, puts it, 'sentience experiences are a cognitive illusion'.

Daniel Dennett is one of the definitive exponents of the modern determinist/physicalist position. In his important book *Consciousness Explained* Dennett (1991) sets out his view of consciousness as an epiphenomenon. He argues that recent neuroscience and psychology, together with experiments in artificial intelligence, enable us to sweep away our traditional view of consciousness. In an argument reminiscent of Hume, he suggests that what people think of as their own stream of consciousness is not a single identifiable unified phenomenon. Rather it represents 'multiple drafts' of reality composed by the biological computer of our brain. Our illusion of consciousness is similar to an experience of virtual reality within a computer game – an epiphenomenon that follows after the computer-generated thing itself.

Both Ryle and Dennett offer us a form of logical argument:

1   The brain is a complex biological machine, whose workings are in principal open to scientific explanation.
2   A physicalist model of the brain is adequate to explain how its input states generate its output states.
3   Therefore consciousness can only be an epiphenomenon.

Modern neuropsychology, following Ryle, deals with the mind/body problem in a simple way – there is no 'strong' conscious mind. That is not to dispute the existence of a *sense impression* of possessing a mind. Rather it is saying that the mind, in the sense of a non-material entity possessing volition, is an illusion or artefact produced as a by-product of the complex activity of the brain. It is a rejection of any strong concept of consciousness, seeing the mind as the epiphe-nomenon of 'mere consciousness'.

The trouble is that every large complex problem has a simple solution – and it's usually wrong. The more we look at physicalist determinism as an answer to the hard problem of consciousness the more difficulties lurk under its attractive façade. Let us look at some of these problems. If we wish to argue for a non-physicalist account of strong consciousness we must question two separate propositions:

Proposition 1: The world is a deterministic machine, therefore the brain must be a deterministic biological machine.

Proposition 2: Physicalism gives us a complete account of the world.

Question 1. Is the world a deterministic machine, and the brain a deterministic biological machine?

Problems with scientific determinism

Determinism is, in its currently fashionable forms, very much the child of early twentieth century modernism. It is hard though not to feel that it has been caught out by history. Nineteenth century science almost had the universe sorted out – an excellent launching pad for determinism and the abolition of the conscious self. But just as the determinist hypothesis was being completed science got weirder. There have been three revolutions in twentieth century science that have made the nice controlled world of determinism look less satisfactory.

Scientific revolutions

At the beginning of the twentieth century, whilst there was plenty of filling in of the gaps still to do, physics at least was all sorted out. Newton's laws were in every possible sense 'true' and unassailable. But in 1905 Einstein published the first of his papers on relativity, and these were confirmed by observations of an eclipse in 1919. In one sense Einstein was only saying that Newton was, under normal terrestrial conditions, slightly wrong. But this is like the teenage girl who protests that she is only slightly pregnant. Newton's world was as chaste and perfect as the celestial spheres of the Middle Ages. To tamper with it was to destroy its significance as Truth with a capital T.

Einstein himself (1959), in a letter to Popper, wrote, 'Observation is theory dependent'. Thus an ancient Greek scientist observes that wood burns, giving off a cloud of smoke and leaving behind ash, supporting his theory that wood is in fact a mixture of earth (the ash) air and fire, supporting the four element model of matter. Popper suggests that we cannot prove theories, but we may be able to disprove them. Thus the four element model did not survive better methods of chemical analysis. After Popper the truth of science was not to be absolute, but provisional. Science can only make claims to a 'best buy' model of reality that is stamped with an unclear sell by date. Karl Popper (1934) stated that 'we cannot identify science with truth'.

Thomas Kuhn (1962) takes this idea one step further. He argues that scientific paradigms do not evolve gracefully as refinements of previous knowledge, but occur as revolutionary events, when enough weight of contradictory observation has discredited a previous paradigm. Furthermore, the weight of evidence needed to endanger an existing paradigm is not determined by scientific logic alone, but also by social and aesthetic influences. 'Reality' is a human construct that will therefore be strongly influenced by cultural and historical perspectives. Facts change at an alarming rate these days.

Quantum theory

It's not just the vast reaches of the universe that have become seriously weird in the twentieth century. Subatomic particles refuse to obey Newton also. Sub-atomic particles are so weird that their properties and relationships can only be modelled in mathematical terms, not described with words. Electrons are both particles and waves. Particles behave differently when observed. We can never know where a particle is at any given moment. There is no particular reason why a particle should not suddenly relocate itself three inches to the left at any given moment. As Niels Bohr (1927) said 'anyone who is not shocked by quantum theory does not understand it'. The behaviour of any individual particle is not *predictable*. Particles are predictable within statistical limits *en masse*, but individually their behaviour is not predictable – they display acausality (Milburn, 1997). Acausality now lies at the centre of orthodox science, welcome or not.

Chaos theory

Chaos theory is better understood as a theory of complexity. Tiny effects build up exponentially due to positive feedback within large systems. In complex systems, infinitesimal variances in a starting point can lead to massive changes in end points (Gleick, 1988). This has been called the butterfly effect – a butterfly flapping its wings could, in theory, lead to a hurricane forming far away. Chaos theory shows that behaviour within complex systems is unpredictable. To make the point clear – not hard to predict but *impossible* to predict. This is not due to indeterminacy, but rather to the overwhelming hugeness and complexity of large systems and the exponential effects of small variances within them. In practical terms this is no different from indeterminacy.

The implications for the brain

The human brain is the most complex object known to man. The human brain contains about 10^{11} neurones (coincidentally about the same number of the stars in our galaxy). Each neurone has thousands of connections with its neighbours. And the firing of an individual signal forming part of a message across the synaptic space between neurones occurs at an order of size where individual quantum effects come into play.

The brain clearly fulfils the criteria for a large complex system that will lack fully predictable outputs. Such a system will function *within* predictable parameters, but its individual actions can never be reliably predicted. Furthermore the brain relies on processes which, at the molecular level, are subject to quantum indeterminacy – to acausality.

Any attempt to show that the brain must function deterministically is pure nineteenth century. If I am to take modern science seriously then the brain possesses the attributes of a machine without determinacy.

One might raise the issue of Haggard's experiment that shows that neural action precedes conscious volition. There are of course a number of problems with this experiment. The most significant is the distinction between choosing overarching goals that we pursue as conscious selves and the more trivial task of executing specific acts. Demonstrating the short subconscious timeline of biological mechanisms leading to specific acts is making only an unimportant point. It would be bizarre to return to a Cartesian model of our *res cogitans* moving our *res extensa* without any intermediate neurological mechanisms. This is not the issue. The issue is whether, within the massive department store that is our brain, there is any thread of control from a conscious self. Haggard's experiment is silent on this point.

But what of our beautiful PET scans, finally showing how the brain is wired up for action? Do these not show us, at last, the brain working as a deterministic machine? This is a misguided claim. We have always known that the brain is wired up internally – the existence of neural functions is not in dispute. We now know more about the wiring in action. This actually tells us nothing about consciousness, only about the wires used to analyse data and execute actions. If we compare it to a telephone system, it certainly tells us who is ringing whom, but nothing about the content of the conversation. And if minds are real it gets us no closer to knowing how minds and brains form part of one whole system.

It is, of course, tempting to go on to speculate that my consciousness gives the odd quantum nudge just at the point where it will have a snowballing effect and change the output at a macroscopic level. But this is to race far beyond any established data. Such a Cartesian interactionist theory is at present fanciful, *and unnecessary*. The determinists such as Ryle were not saying they knew how the brain worked, forcing us to offer a counter theory. They were simply saying that by the best available knowledge of the time the brain *must* be a deterministic system. But twenty-first century science no longer preaches physical determinism within large complex systems that rely on many small active components. A deterministic brain is no longer a given. Therefore physicalism cannot claim that it *must* be true. To be credible, physicalism must demonstrate that it leaves nothing out of its description of the world. Let us see if this is so.

Question 2: Does physicalism give us a complete account of the world?

Strong subjectivity

By a physicalist account, our consciousness is only an epiphenomenon of the biological functions of our brain. This is the conceptual backdrop of an impoverished view of persons now promoted by many contemporary neuroscientists and some philosophers. But an impoverished view of the human condition forms the intellectual backdrop for an impoverished evidence base and an impoverished and impersonal medical practice. But is it true?

Physicalism cannot be true if we find that it leaves anything out of a comprehensive description of the universe that we actually experience. So if the mind is indeed an epiphenomenon, then physicalism might give us a complete picture of the known universe. But if there is persuasive evidence that we cannot completely explain the mind in physical terms then physicalism cannot be a complete model of the universe.

Physicalism relies upon the empirical method. Essentially physicalism's claim is that of 'positivism' – only what can be measured by science counts. But why? Science is a brilliant way of knowing about matter-energy within space-time. But science can have no up-front claim that there can be *nothing except* matter-energy within space-time. The real question is, what reason might we have for models that go beyond matter-energy within space-time? We would need some persuasive arguments for a non-physicalist model. But we cannot initially accept that *only* physicalism might be true.

Physicalism is rejected by many philosophers, both historic and contemporary. They claim that consciousness cannot be reduced to physical processes in the material world. Materialist theories of mind omit the essential component of consciousness, namely that there is something that it feels like to be a particular conscious thing. There are two essential elements that form an argument, not from observing things *outside* ourselves via empiricism, but from *inside* ourselves, via subjectivity.

First we must understand what we mean here by subjectivity. We are used to treating subjectivity as second class: 'I think that picture is really lovely.' 'No, that's just your subjective opinion, I think it's too sentimental.' This is not the subjectivity to which I am referring. By subjectivity I am referring to the internal awareness and sense perceptions that we experience directly within our conscious minds. In other words, we are observers, not just observed. And perhaps authors, not only readers. I cannot measure the content of my consciousness. You certainly cannot measure my subjective experiences, as my consciousness has no connection to your consciousness. I must first externalize my experiences and then convey them by communication such as speech. Thus there exists a privileged 'space' within myself where I am aware of my own existence and where I am aware of my own experiences.

David Chalmers puts it like this:

> Consciousness is a surprising feature of our universe. Our grounds for believing in consciousness derive solely from our own experience of it. Even if we knew every last detail about the physics of the universe ... *that* information would not lead us to postulate the existence of conscious experience.... It is my first-person experience of consciousness that forces the problem on me.
>
> (1996, p. 101)

Chalmers (1996) outlines the hard problem by asking 'why does the feeling which accompanies awareness of sensory information exist at all?' He argues that there is an *explanatory gap* from the objective to the subjective.

Science gives us probabilistically reliable ways of modelling and manipulating matter-energy within space-time, but we should not confuse this with reliable knowledge of the world itself, except in a partial and instrumental sense. What access might we have to knowledge of the world itself? Surely all access must start via our senses. And here we find our senses start with an immediate self-awareness before all else. The first thing I experience when I awake in the morning is myself, or to be more accurate, an awareness of my own self-aware mind. Thomas Nagel states:

> I have argued that the seductive appeal of objective reality depends on a mistake. It is not the given. Reality is not just objective reality. Sometimes in the philosophy of the mind but also elsewhere, the truth is not to be found by travelling as far away from one's personal perspective as possible.
>
> (1986, p. 27)

There are two types of experience for which we can claim this ultimate subjectivity. The most fundamental is my own self-awareness – I am *aware* that I am. This is unmediated and unmeasurable. I have no reason to believe that a stone or a computer has an awareness of itself (although as we do not know what makes minds happen it is possible that a computer may have self-awareness in the future). Technically I cannot even know for certain that other persons possess self-aware consciousness – I can only infer it from their statements that they have and from the general implausibility of solipsism (philosophers refer to this as 'the problem of other minds' – a problem whose insolubility troubled me as a child). I raise this as it illustrates my need, if I am to make sense of the world, to rely on reasons other than direct observation and 'scientific proofs'. I also have to ask what makes most sense! (It is reasonable to suppose that some other animals, such as chimps, dolphins and elephants, may possess self-aware consciousness, but this is not directly relevant here.)

The other element of strong subjectivity is what are termed 'qualia' (Misselbrook, 2014, p. 248). Qualia are the immediate internal sensations derived from perception, such as 'redness', or pain, prior to us processing them within conceptual models. How do I know that the redness I perceive when I look at a pillar box is the same as the redness you perceive? An exhaustive physical description of the perception of red objects does not contain an account of the qualia I experience as 'redness'. Frank Jackson (1982) argues that if physical science can tell us all that can be known, then a colour blind person must be able to know what it is to see red. We can construct this knowledge around a model of having the right sort of cones in the retina to perceive incident light with a wavelength of 650 nm etc. Yet if this person – in possession of all available knowledge *about* redness – were to be cured of their colour blindness then they will learn something new that they did not know before – what it is to see red. An exhaustive physical description of the perception of red objects does not contain an account of the qualia I experience as 'redness'. Jackson's argument is a demonstration of something that is both profound and also obvious to all but the most extreme physicalist. Qualia, and thus human self-awareness, cannot be contained within a purely physical account of the self.

There is a secondary sense in which strong subjectivity is also a relevant issue – that of broader personalistic knowledge (Polanyi, 1998). This is of less relevance to us philosophically as it does not relate to the possibility of physicalism being an inadequate explanation for the mind. However, it illustrates that scientific knowledge is not our fundamental concern as humans. Unless one takes an extreme physicalist or reductionist position, empirically verifiable facts are not the only species of reality to be found in the world that we live in. Erwin Schrödinger made this point well:

> The scientific picture of the world around me is very deficient. It gives me a lot of factual information, puts all our experience in a magnificently consistent order, but is ghastly silent about all that is really near to our heart, that really matters to us. It cannot tell a word about the sensation of red and blue, bitter and sweet … it knows nothing of beauty and ugly, good or bad…. Science sometimes pretends to answer questions in these domains, but the answers are so silly that we are not inclined to take them seriously.
>
> (1964, p. 93)

Beyond physicalism?

By a physicalist account we are operated by our animal pre-conscious minds but have developed something we perceive as self-awareness, that we mistakenly interpret as being in control. Such physicalism is attractive for a number of reasons. It is simple. All we need is matter-energy located within space-time and we have described the universe, including ourselves. Second there is still no convincing solution to the mind/body problem, the so called hard problem. But if we eliminate the category of mind (in the strong sense) we have solved the mind/

body problem – a result. Third our recent successes have been in the sciences (they have certainly not been in the moral world). It's satisfying to stick to what you're good at.

But we have seen that physicalism does not adequately model the world itself. It is only making the best of a bad job following a wrong assumption of matter-energy within space-time being the only *possible* valid categories. But there are always brute facts in any world. We cannot explain the existence of matter-energy or of space-time. They are brute facts. We cannot explain the existence of natural laws – more brute facts. Similarly we are unlikely to explain scientifically why the world contains minds, however, if we have good reason to believe they exist, we may reasonably accept them as brute facts also. It is reasonable to believe minds could not exist without a physical world to support them, even though minds are not needed for a physical world to exist. Physical descriptions do not always tell the whole story. It would be unreasonable to insist that there is no such thing as 'a symphony' on my CD because science can only identify a piece of plastic with microscopic indentations arranged in a particular way. Higher order realities may attain their own status as real entities in the world.

So, there is something about consciousness that cannot be reduced down to physical processes in the material world. Consciousness is often seen as an 'emergent' quality. In a large complex system (such as a brain) qualities, indeed realities, 'emerge' that are more than the sum of their lower-order constituent parts. But there is another side to emergent qualities. A more important model is that of supervenience (Chalmers, 1996, Chapter 3). In a large complex system higher order B-properties may supervene – that is they can be fully explained – by lower order A-properties. Thus we know how cells pass on their performance characteristics (B-properties) by reference to the biochemistry of DNA replication plus epigenetic phenomena (A-properties). And we know how DNA replication works (now B-properties) by reference to the basic biochemical models of atomic bonds and enzyme function (A-properties) etc. In this chain of examples the lower order properties, starting with atomic structure and atomic bonds, determine higher order structures by logical necessity. They determine what sort of cells will work and what will not. Yet, not only is consciousness *not* a necessity for brain function (as Dennett strains to remind us) but consciousness does not supervene logically on the physical. Whilst it seems clear that the mind needs the brain in order for it to exist there is nothing within physicalism that makes consciousness a necessary outcome of a physicalist interpretation of brain function; i.e. the functioning brain could exist without the mind. The mind does not *have* to exist – and yet it is there.

Why accept strong consciousness?

There are certain irreducible foundational truths. Why should I believe that I exist within an actual world instead of Plato's cave or the Wachowski siblings'

Matrix? (These two examples are more formally represented by Gilbert Harman's (1973, p. 5) 'brain in a vat' thought experiment, contested by Hillary Putnam.) Again, why should I believe in the existence of other minds? You cannot *prove* that they are there. And yet a reasonable person would accept some unprovable things as overwhelmingly probable. So I do not believe in the existence of an external world and the existence of other minds because they have been proven, but as a *best explanation* of things. This is called 'inference to the best explanation' (ITBE) and is commonly seen as the best defence against strong scepticism, and as the most reliable way of deciding between competing theories (Harman, 1965). ITBE gives us no guarantee of truth, however to expect such a guarantee would be unreasonable as we have no God's eye view of the world as our guarantor. In appealing to ITBE we are using a particular knowledge seeking practice not because we believe we can be certain, but because we have no better method to hand (i.e. we use ITBE not from an a priori commitment but for its a posteriori instrumental value).

Physicalism is a man-made model of the world, not some self-evident truth. It commonly takes the form of rather circular logic which I can perhaps parody as follows:

Premise 1: Science is our best way of knowing.

(Opel et al., 2011)

Premise 2: Science can only detect matter-energy phenomena within space-time.
Conclusion: Therefore only matter-energy phenomena within space-time exist.

The problem is that the initial premise can only be argued by accepting the conclusion as one's starting point. However, science is a human activity. It may well be our best method of modelling matter-energy objects existing within space-time, however it has no up-front guarantee of providing a complete model of the world itself. We would be justified in believing it may be complete if we can find nothing left out, but not otherwise. And we have seen what physicalism leaves out.

How can we build a better model?

We must return to basic theories of knowledge. If we reject the simple model offered by physicalism our progress is limited by two factors. The first is an empirical problem – our lack of knowledge of the ultimate natures of matter and mind. The second is a conceptual problem – the 'noumenon/phenomenon' problem, which I shall explain. This has been restated in various ways throughout history, from Plato's (381 BC) Theory of Forms, through St Paul's (AD 53–57) *'seeing through a glass darkly'* (I Corinthians 13:12) to Kant's more explicit account. Immanuel Kant argued that:

As the senses never enable us to know things in themselves, but only their appearances, all bodies must be held to be nothing but mere representations in us, and exist nowhere else than merely in our thought.

(Kant, 1783, section 13, note II)

Kant explained that we have no direct knowledge of the world itself. We construct models of the world in our mind from our perceptions. Kant (1781, part II section I) also argued that *observations without theories are blind* (my paraphrase). He means we cannot make use of any individual observation in building a picture of the world unless we can fit that observation into some theoretical framework which we ourselves construct. So, as a doctor, if I see a Cusco speculum I see it *as* a Cusco speculum, but a non-medic would just see it as a weird duck-billed metal instrument. And what I see as a chipped old stone my remote ancestors would immediately recognise as a carefully crafted hand axe. Hick (1989), after Wittgenstein, understands this as *experiencing-as*, and goes so far as to say that 'all seeing is seeing-as; or rather that all conscious experiencing, including seeing, is experiencing-as' (p. 140). So we are left with a two-step knowledge system that will depend upon individual observations of the world which we fit into man-made models or theory systems.

All knowledge must be held in the form of hypotheses, and all knowledge models must be seen only as models within Popper's fallibilist framework. If they are successful we may claim them as a current best-buy model of reality. However to claim any model as complete would be unwarranted.

We have already agreed that empiricism may be the most reliable knowledge seeking practice for the construction of knowledge about matter-energy within space-time. But let us remember there are also necessary truths, such as mathematics. $1+1=2$ needs no empirical verification – it is a necessary truth. Necessary truths exist without the need of any specific observations to support them.

Wilfred Sellars (1962) argues that *ways* of thinking are prior to scientific thinking. Empiricism is a method of seeking knowledge, clearly successful in modelling the physical world but with no a priori guarantee of giving us access to the world as it is in itself. Mary Midgely (2014a) points out that science tells us apparently solid tables are mostly empty space but that does not mean we should stop putting our coffee cups on them. 'Just as we can accommodate more than one way of thinking about tables so we can accommodate more than one way of thinking about ourselves. A unifying theory is unnecessary.' I commend Midgely's defense of the conscious mind and would echo her argument that: 'thoughts have their real place among other kinds of causes in the world.... Minds can affect brains as well as brains affecting minds' (Midgley, 2014, p. 104).

Thus whilst we might agree that a physicalist model suits very well for the physics of hitting tennis balls or sending up spacecraft there is no reason for us to be bound by its self-validating logic as a universal guarantor for what is or is not allowed to exist. Physicalism is a human model that has no a priori claim to truth. As a human model it may be expected to have its limitations. So does physicalism adequately represent the world that we actually experience? If it does not then we must seek a better model.

Neuroscience and strong consciousness may make uneasy bedfellows, but, in the real universe, the universe in part revealed to us by science, they may well be apparently mutually incompatible and yet both true. The problem turns out to be one of language and models, not one of fact. In the twenty-first century matter and energy are inextricably linked, and space and time are inextricably linked – there is no apparent *logical* necessity to have both these essential elements of the world. They are both brute facts, or as Bertrand Russell (1919, p. 182) put it, they are both part of the furniture of the world. Chalmers (1996, p. 214) cites consciousness as part of the furniture of the world in just the same sense. It is a brute fact, irreducible to simpler parts.

Towards an integrated self

Certainly we do not yet have the data (or is it just the language?) for a unifying theory of neuroscience and strong consciousness. But current physicalist theories cannot claim to have banished strong consciousness. There are enough grounds, both from our knowledge systems and from our own direct experience, to take consciousness seriously, therefore rumours of its death should be seen as greatly exaggerated.

Let me appeal again to the analogy of the electron. We know the world is weird at a subatomic (or ultimate) level. It is not the case that an electron is half particle and half wave, nor it is the case that it is sometimes one and sometimes the other. It is not a bit of each but is fully both at the same time. Whether we perceive it as particle or wave depends on what properties we are observing. It depends on our viewpoint, and on the model within which we are working. It is no good, in the name of reason, to give an ultimatum to the electron that it must make up its mind and plump for one existence or the other. An electron itself is as it is, and it up to us to model it as best we may.

Why then shouldn't our brains be 'merely' physical organs yet strong consciousness also real? This surely will depend upon the model being used and the language with which we construct such models. If we accept Einstein's view that observation is theory dependent then this implies that the perception, interpretation and use of data is dependent upon the paradigm or model within which we are seeing that data.

Of course, it is possible that quantum mechanics and relativity will be reconciled into a unified 'theory of everything'. Einstein was unable to accomplish this, and no less a figure than Hawking (1998, Chapter 10) has so far failed in our generation. Such a theory would presumably give us a unified model of the electron, which will encompass and supersede its current dual nature status.

Similarly there have been those, such as William James and Bertrand Russell, who have maintained that the mind body problem will ultimately turn out to be a non-problem. Perhaps we will devise a more adequate theory that, instead of positing a ghost in the machine, or throwing out the ghost and leaving just machine, will accommodate both 'ghost' and machine in synthesis.

Neuroscience without physicalism?

Chalmers states:

> if consciousness cannot be reductively explained … we … need to move to a *nonreductive* theory instead. We can give up on the project of trying to explain the existence of consciousness wholly in terms of something more basic, and instead admit it as fundamental, giving an account of how it relates to everything else in the world.
>
> (1996, p. 213)

Science does not tell us all we need to know. Mary Midgley (2014) states: 'Science is unfortunately not composed of ready-made facts. People who formulate those facts have to use assumptions: patterns of expectation, within which they select, arrange, shape and classify their data.' Midgley describes her 'increasing exasperation at … many well qualified scholars to claim, apparently in the name of science, that they believe themselves, and indeed their readers, not to exist, selves having apparently been replaced by arrangements of brain cells' (p. 141). True models may overlap even where they appear incompatible. We can accommodate more than one way of thinking about ourselves. A unifying theory between neuroscience and strong consciousness is not necessary.

So let us re-examine two of Ryle's accusations. First he argues that: 'the physical world is a deterministic system, *so* the mental world must be a deterministic system. Bodies cannot help the modifications that they undergo, *so* minds cannot help pursing the careers fixed for them' (1949, Chapter III, 2 [my italics]). We can clearly see that his statements rely on an initial presumption of physicalism – he begs the question. If minds are real then why should they follow the same rules as the physical world?

Second we noted that Ryle describes Descartes concept of mind as 'the ghost in the machine', a category error that wrongly insists that 'minds are not bits of clockwork, they are just bits of non-clockwork'. It is not necessary for us to have a fully worked up model of what mind is 'made of' in order to refute Ryle. It is only necessary for us to establish the validity of 'mind' as a real category in the world. 'Mind stuff' is a project in hand, just as explaining how relativity and quantum mechanics exist within the same world is a project in hand. Chalmers (1996, p. 215) points out the difficulties that face us in seeking to construct a robust model of consciousness as 'consciousness is not directly observable in experimental contexts'. This, of course, is the point – we are the subject, not the object; the observer, not the observed.

We may not have even begun to start to map out this mountain, but at least we have noticed that it is there. As Chalmers (1996, p. 3) says: 'We know consciousness far more intimately than we know the rest of the world, but we understand the rest of the world far better than we understand consciousness'.

So what?

Let us revisit our three patients from the perspective of their inner subjectivity.

Due to his current academic studies, James sees his problem as biochemical. We are likely to see his problem as an assault on his personal relationships, hopes and plans due to a violent rupture in an intimate and committed relationship that had formed a central part of his self-identity. Furthermore we may well feel that influencing James' thoughts is more likely to be beneficial than influencing his neurotransmitters. If we can help James to process his painful thoughts then his brain biochemistry is likely to follow. We will wish to negotiate with James and to work with him on this one.

Edith Brown presents us with a series of biomedical problems to be managed. Yet her internal world is far richer but more challenging than her list of biomedical problems. Can our gaze include her subjective world? A world with rich memories, yet present existential trials. Mrs Brown challenges us to consider the proper goals of medicine. Her body is challenged but has the potential to be stabilised. The way we approach this task is likely to either limit or extend her freedom. So what should take priority, our 'objective' biomedical goals or her 'subjective' life goals, that exist only within her conscious mind? What is most important to us?

Mrs Sayyid has obvious problems with her brain function. We have some partly worked out models of the brain in dementia, but not enough to reverse the process for her. But clearly she has a very active inner life. We have a problem with this as, from our perspective, it is partly delusional. Her situation reminds me of Édouard Manet's picture of *The Execution of Emperor Maximilian*, in the National Gallery. The original picture has been cut into several pieces, with some sections lost. Yet what remains, although incomplete, remains a masterpiece. With some effort we can work out its meaning. It remains a work of richness and great worth. Yet this richness and worth, again, only exists within Mrs Sayyid's conscious mind. Until we have definitive treatments it is her self-aware consciousness that matters most, not the biomedical model of the failing organ that is her brain. So can we engage with Mrs Sayyid, the conscious self-aware human whose brain malfunction has left her coping with a partly delusional world view? Can we engage with the parts of her inner world that would enable her to flourish, despite this cognitive disability? Can we value the parts that are still there and see what picture they paint, even if we have to fill in the blanks? Do we value the personhood still present in Mrs Sayyid's conscious mind?

Conclusion

Physicalism fails as a complete explanation of the world. We are also right to reject Descartes' crude interactionism. We are still on the early stages of a road that might, or might not, solve the 'hard problem' of consciousness. But there is no reason for us to accept the wrong answers of naïve physicalism and determinism. We have every reason to believe the evidence of our own immediate self-awareness and its implication for a strong model of human consciousness. In rejecting physicalist explanations of the mind, we accept the dignity and responsibility of our own status as humans and we affirm the dignity and worth of others, in particular our patients.

Key learning points

1   There is no satisfactory explanation for the nature of human consciousness, or how it relates to the brain as a physical organ. There are two main approaches to this problem.
2   One approach sees consciousness as a by-product of the brain that does not itself affect the brain. We are passengers, not drivers, in our journey through the world. This is termed 'mere consciousness'.
3   The other approach holds that there are reasons to believe that the mind may affect the brain as well as the brain affecting the mind. This is called 'strong consciousness'.
4   Mere consciousness assumes that, in principle, the brain must be a predictable machine and that a physical description of the world can explain everything that we observe.
5   Strong consciousness argues that the brain may not have the characteristics of a predictable machine and that a purely physical explanation of the world may not explain everything that we observe.
6   We are not yet in a position to give a comprehensive theory of strong consciousness.
7   There are however good scientific and philosophical reasons to defend the possibility of strong consciousness.
8   These issues matter if we wish to put the personhood of the patient at the heart of medical practice.

References

Bohr, N. 1927. As quoted in Barad, K. 2007. *Meeting the universe halfway*. Durham NC, Duke University Press, p. 254.
Chalmers, D. 1995. 'Facing up to the problem of consciousness'. *Journal of Consciousness Studies*, 2 (3): 200–19.
Chalmers, D. 1996. *The Conscious Mind: In Search of a Fundamental Theory*. Oxford: Oxford University Press.
Dennett, D. 1991. *Consciousness explained*. Boston: Little Brown and Co.
Descartes, R. 1641. *Meditations*.
Einstein, A. 1934. Einstein's letter to Popper, quoted as appendix to '*Logic der Forschung*' 1934, translated as *The logic of scientific discovery*. London: Hutchinson, 1959.
Gleick, J. 1988. *Chaos*. London: Heinemann.
Haggard, P., Newman, C. and Magno, E. 1999. On the perceived time of voluntary actions. *British Journal of Psychology*, 90: 291–303.
Harman, G. 1965. The Inference to the Best Explanation. *Philosophical Review*, 74: 88–95.
Harman, G. 1973. *Thought*. New Jersey: Princeton University Press.

118   *D. Misselbrook*

Hawking, S. 1998. *A brief history of time*. London: Bantam Press.

Hick, J. 1989. *An interpretation of religion*. Basingstoke: Macmillan Press.

Hume, D. 1739. *A treatise of human nature*.

Huxley, T. 1874. On the Hypothesis that Animals are Automata, and its History, *The Fortnightly Review* 16 (New Series): 555–80. Reprinted in *Method and Results: Essays by Thomas H. Huxley*. New York: D. Appleton and Company, 1898.

Jackson, F. 1982. Epiphenomenal Qualia. *Philosophical Quarterly*, 32 (127): 127–36.

Kant, I. 1781 (1993). *Critique of pure reason*. London: Everyman.

Kant, I. 1783. *Prolegomena to any future metaphysics*. Section 13, note II.

Kuhn, T. 1962. *The structure of scientific revolutions*. Chicago: University of Chicago.

Midgley, M. 2014. *Are you an illusion?* London: Routledge.

Milburn, G. 1997. *Schrodinger's machines: the quantum technology reshaping everyday life*. New York: W.H. Freeman.

Misselbrook, D. 2014. Q is for Qualia. *BJGP*, 64 (622).

Misselbrook, D. 2015. Aristotle, Hume and the goals of medicine. *Journal of Evaluation in Clinical Practice*, 22 (4): 544–9.

Misselbrook, D. 2016. Book review: The Soul of the Marionette: A Short Enquiry Into Human Freedom. And: Are You An Illusion? *BJGP*, 66: 642.

Nagel, T. 1974. 'What Is It Like to Be a Bat?' *The Philosophical Review,* 83 (4): 435–50.

Nagel, T. 1986. *The view from nowhere*. Oxford: Oxford University Press, p. 27.

Opel, D., Diekema, D. and Marcuse, E. 2011. Assuring research integrity in the wake of Wakefield. *BMJ*, 342: 179–80.

Plato. 381 BC. *The republic*. Book VII.

Polanyi, M. 1958. *Personal knowledge: towards a post-critical philosophy*. First published 1958, republished by Routledge 1998.

Popper, K. 1934 (1959). *Logic der forschung*, translated as *The logic of scientific discovery*. London: Hutchinson.

Ryle, G. 1949. *The concept of mind*. Hutchinson. Reprinted by Penguin, London, 1963.

Russell, B. 1919. *Introduction to mathematical philosophy*. London: G. Allen & Unwin.

Saint Paul. AD 53–57. *The Bible*.

Schrödinger, E. 1964. *My view of the world*. Cambridge: Cambridge University Press.

Sellars, W. 1962. Philosophy and the Scientific Image of Man. *In:* Robert Colodny (ed.) *Frontiers of science and philosophy*. Pittsburgh: University of Pittsburgh Press: 35–78. Reprinted in *Science, perception and reality* (1963).

Weiskrantz, L. 1990. *Blindsight: a case study and implications*. Oxford: Clarendon Press.

6 Patient, person, self

Christopher Dowrick

Introduction

There is a fundamental need for a concept of the self which provides all patients with dignity and respect during their encounters in primary health care.

In this chapter I will explain how the concept of the self which I originally proposed in the context of depression might – after some revisions – meet this need. I will also consider its practical application, in clinical encounters between primary health care professionals and their patients.

Coherence, engagement and depression

I begin with a summary of my concept of the self in relation to the experience of depression (Dowrick, 2009, 2016), which is based on the two principal components of coherence and engagement.

Coherence

I advocate an understanding of ourselves as coherent beings, neither wholly individualised on the one hand, nor illusory, fragmented or role-playing on the other hand; and within this an understanding of ourselves as persons with agency, with the capacity to lead our own lives. This is based on the assumption that human life has an essential unity throughout its whole extent, that we are fundamentally real and intrinsically valuable beings, who have the capacity to change and progress.

I suggest that our coherence is based on four important elements: desire, memory, imagination and curiosity.

Desire refers to our innate will to persist and continue with our lives; it articulates our dogged determination to survive, come what may. Desire is apparent in literature, for example with the '*life hungry stupidity*' of Pi, when faced with the prospect of sharing a lifeboat with a Royal Bengal tiger:

> We fight no matter the cost of the battle, the losses we take, the improbability of success. We fight to the very end. It is not a question of courage. It's something constitutional, an inability to let go. It may be nothing more than life-hungry stupidity.
>
> (Martel, 2002, p. 148)

Our desire to survive is also apparent in life, for example with Joe Simpson's response to falling onto a precarious ice bridge inside a vast Andean crevasse:

> The idea of waiting alone and maddened for so long had forced me to this choice: abseil until I could find a way out, or die in the process. I would meet it rather than wait for it to come to me.
>
> (Simpson, 1997, p. 130)

My understanding of this concept of desire as the essence of our being derives from the *conatus* of Baruch Spinoza, the seventeenth century Dutch philosopher. Spinoza proposed that 'the desire by which each thing desires to persevere in its being is nothing other than *the actual essence of the thing* [my emphasis]'. He further asserts that 'the mind, both in so far as it has clear and distinct ideas and in so far as it has confused ideas, desires in its being for an indefinite duration, and is conscious of this desire' (Spinoza, 2000). We will return to Spinoza's *conatus* later, when considering how even confused minds can have continuous consciousness.

Memory is the principal means by which we demonstrate our sense of continuity to ourselves, linking thoughts and emotions in a way that produces a sense of self-coherence (Wollheim, 1984). For the French novelist Marcel Proust, the interaction between sensation and memory – most famously described in his story of the piece of madeleine soaked in a cup of tea – is the key to his sense of self and his wellbeing:

> And at once the vicissitudes of life had become indifferent to me, its disasters innocuous, its brevity illusory – this new sensation having had the effect, which love has, of filling me with a precious essence; or rather this essence was not in me, *it was me*. I had ceased now to feel mediocre, contingent, mortal.
>
> (Proust, 2002, p. 51 [my emphasis])

We can turn memory into a source of energy, either by drawing new implications from old memories or else by expansion, incorporating the experiences of others (Zeldin, 1994).

Curiosity refers to our eagerness to find out about new things, our inquisitiveness, our sense of excitement at finding the unexpected. In 350 BC Aristotle introduced his Metaphysics with the statement 'All men by nature desire to know' (Ross, 1953). Descartes (1967) agrees: our innate curiosity is an essential means of increasing knowledge. Zeldin (1994) takes this argument a stage further. Reflecting on the life of Alexander von Humboldt, he concludes that curiosity can be a successful remedy against sadness and fear. If we use our personal worries as stimuli to explore the general mystery of the universe 'the limits of curiosity are at the frontiers of despair'.

Imagination is the ability to produce ideas or images of what is not present or has not been experienced, and the ability to deal creatively with unexpected or unusual problems. The enhancement of memory by imagination can help us 'through the traffic jams of the brain' (Zeldin, 1994, pp. 441–2). Imagination is liberating when it is constructive, arranging fertile marriages between images and sensations, recombining obstacles to make them useful, spotting what is both unique and universal in them.

Engagement

The second component of my original concept of the self was the assumption that we make sense of ourselves and find meaning in our engagement with the world around us: in the context of the history, places or 'practices' within which we find ourselves, and which we have the ability to modify; and within this, a belief that such engagement – whether constructed in political, social or personal terms – is crucial in creating our sense of identity and well-being.

Our sense of identity has important social dimensions. Language and culture are important in defining and shaping our understanding of emotional states. They are also highly relevant to understanding ourselves.

Engagement may take the form of participation in practices and moral communities, in 'coherent and socially established cooperative human activity' with inherent standards of excellence (MacIntyre, 1984): in this sense it is closely related to the Greek term *eudaemonia*, which encompasses both *being* well and *doing* well. Practices involve the use of a set of skills in a systematic way, with the intention of enriching our lives and the lives of those around us. They may be self-contained, such as chess, music or sport; or purposive, such as law and politics. Moral communities involve friendship within common pursuit of purposes beyond oneself, such as the political community of classical Athens, medieval monastic orders or the liberation movements in late twentieth century Africa.

Engagement may take the simpler form, proposed by Charles Taylor, of the affirmation of ordinary life through investment in our networks, our 'webs of interlocution':

> in the family tree, in social space, in the geography of social statuses and functions, in my intimate relations to the ones I love, and also crucially in the space of moral and spiritual orientation within which my most important defining relations are lived out.
>
> (Taylor, 1984, p. 36)

Engagement may also take the form of commitment to the circumstances in which we find ourselves, whatever they may be, whether they involve cultural alienation or physical illness, and our determination to make of them the best we can. Our role model here is the boulder-pushing Sisyphus, as interpreted by Albert Camus. For Camus, the struggle to survive against overwhelming odds, as we strain to push our boulders up the mountain every day, is sufficient cause for happiness: '*La lutte elle-même vers les sommets suffit à remplir un cœur d'homme. Il faut imaginer Sisyphe heureux'* (Camus, 1942). My translation of this is: 'The struggle towards the heights is, in itself, enough to fill a man's heart. We need to imagine that Sisyphus is happy.'

Usefulness for depression

My original intention in setting out this strong concept of the self, in proposing that we are persons with the capacity to lead our lives, was quite practical. I wanted to reinterpret the depressive state and (in so doing) offer alternative routes out of it, based on understanding and meaning-making rather than on diagnosis and treatment.

There is evidence emerging in support of the usefulness of this concept for people with experience of depression. A weak sense of coherence is predictive of the onset of depressive disorders (Lehtinen *et al.*, 2005), while conversely, identifying our strengths and using them in new ways can reduce depressive symptoms (Seligman *et al.*, 2005). Depressed people with positive illness beliefs have improved outcomes (Lynch *et al.*, 2015). People who adopt strategies of personal resilience, taking steps to build personal strengths and expand positive emotions, recover more quickly from depressive episodes than those who do not (Griffiths *et al.*, 2015).

Coherence, engagement and long term conditions

I now propose that the concept of the coherent, engaged self has broader validity and utility in contemporary primary health care. I think it can be applied to the great majority of patients whom we encounter in our consultations, including those living with multi-morbidity and long term conditions. It provides an underpinning for our emphasis on shared decision-making, and the expectations placed upon us – whether on ethical or on economic grounds – to encourage patient self-management.

Mechanical metaphors

As Stefán Hjörleifsson, Kjersti Lea and David Misselbrook discuss elsewhere in this book, medicine's basis in the physical sciences leads clinicians in primary care to adopt concepts of the patient self which are passive and mechanistic.

John Skelton and colleagues, in an analysis of the metaphors used in routine primary care consultations, demonstrated that GPs tend to use mechanical metaphors to explain diseases. They consider patients' problems as puzzles, and cast themselves in the roles of problem solvers and controllers of disease. When talking about psychological unease, GPs tend to use words based on the physical metaphors of tension and relaxation, speaking about problems to do with nerves and the nervous system, and about ways in which medication may affect a finely balanced system (Skelton *et al.*, 2002).

But there is a fundamental flaw with this perspective. It puts the onus on doctors to achieve change, while undermining patients' sense of enablement. It is a recipe for burnout for the doctor and failure for the patient. It contradicts our stated intentions of promoting patient self-management, joint decision-making (Farrelly *et al.*, 2015) and 'shared mind' (Epstein and Street, 2011; Epstein, 2013). It squeezes both doctor and patient into a suffocating conceptual cul-de-sac.

Long term conditions

The concept of a coherent, engaged self has potential benefit for people living with diabetes, heart disease and other chronic health problems, whether as single or multi-morbid conditions. It provides a new set of metaphors, dynamic and temporal rather than passive and deterministic, with concepts of personhood and the self which contain possibilities of hope, action and purpose.

It offers my patient Ken a basis on which to define himself positively, to tell good stories about himself and (if he so wishes) to participate actively with health professionals in managing his condition.

Ken is 67 and has chronic obstructive pulmonary disease. He has to stop for breath after walking about 100 metres, which is grade of four (out of five) on the MRC breathlessness scale. His forced expiratory volume is 48 per cent of predicted normal, putting him into the severe (GOLD 3) category. His oxygen saturation varies between 85 per cent and 88 per cent. He uses a combination of long-acting and short-acting bronchodilators and an inhaled steroid, with supplementary oxygen especially at night. He also has benign prostatic hyperplasia and essential hypertension, which are reasonably controlled with alpha and calcium channel blockers, and episodes of gastritis for which he takes a proton pump inhibitor.

Ken worked for years on the Liverpool docks, loading and unloading everything under the sun, with constant exposure to dust and various unknown chemicals. As a trade unionist he took part in the long-running dock strike in the mid-1990s, and has many tales to tell about this. After he was laid off, he used his redundancy money to buy into a bar in the city centre.

Ken lives with his wife Lizzy, and his two grown-up daughters are just a few streets away with their own families. He smoked regularly since his early teens, though he's given up now he has to have oxygen at home. He still likes a few cans of beer at home, with the occasional whisky chaser. He used to own racing pigeons, but had to stop as they were affecting his breathing. Most days he enjoys a bet or two on the horses, and wins more than he loses.

He is part of a class action against the Liverpool Docks and Harbour Board, claiming occupational damage to his lungs. He doesn't hold out much hope of success but tells me it would be great for Lizzy if something comes from it eventually, especially after he's gone.

Ken's life these days is comparable to the endless rock-rolling of Camus' Sisyphus. He faces relentless physical pressures to breathe effectively enough to climb the stairs to his bedroom each evening and – on good days – to walk the 200 metres to his local newsagent's to pick up his copy of *Sporting Life*. But he is, usually, defiantly, happy that he has achieved another day. He knows he could move his bed down to the living room, and Lizzy would gladly go out to buy his paper for him but, as he tells me 'I'll show the bastards, there's still plenty of puff in these bloody lungs of mine'. With Spinoza, he is determined to keep on going, come what may.

Sometimes, especially in the depth of the night, Ken joins Heidegger (1996) in confronting his personhood and mortality, in reflecting on the paradox of living in relationship with other humans while being ultimately alone with himself and his illness. He contemplates the meaning of his existence, his past, his personal and cultural history, and an open series of possibilities that he can seize hold of – or not. 'What the fuck, Prof.,' he says, 'I never thought I'd end up like this. But I've still a bloody good life, me family is great, and I do love them horses.'

When he talks like this, he is authentically engaged in the messy, intersubjective coherence of his *Dasein*, his being-in-the-world.

Usefulness for long term conditions

These concepts of coherence and engagement are not just of theoretical interest. They also have practical applications for our health. I will now explain how they may help people who are living with long terms conditions.

For Anton Antonovsky (1987, p. 18), our sense of coherence has three components: a sense of comprehensibility; a sense of manageability; and a sense of meaningfulness. Defined in these terms, a strong sense of coherence is directly correlated with adaptation to chronic obstructive pulmonary disease, contributing significantly to reduced anxiety, depression and disease-specific disability (Keil *et al.*, 2016). Sense of coherence is protective against mortality and functional decline in older people (Boeckxstaens *et al.*, 2016) and mediates their experience of pain (Wiesmann *et al.*, 2014). It predicts quality of life and coping strategies in people living with Parkinson's disease (Pusswald *et al.*, 2012), and emerged as a significant contribution to health-related quality of life for multimorbid primary care patients in Germany (Vogel *et al.*, 2012).

On the other hand, a weak sense of coherence predicted the onset of diabetes in a high risk Norwegian population (Nilsen *et al.*, 2015). It is also associated with a general increase in risk of mortality: a longitudinal study of more than 12,000 adults in the Netherlands found weak sense of coherence predicted 27 per cent higher all-cause risk of mortality (Super *et al.*, 2014); while in England a similar study of over 18,000 adults found a 20 per cent increased risk of all-cause mortality (Wainwright *et al.*, 2008).

Importantly, our sense of coherence is not a static set of personal attributes. It can change over time, and as the result of therapeutic interventions such as mind-body therapies (Fenros *et al.*, 2008), and salutogenic group therapy focusing on inner feelings, immediate personal relations, major activity and existential issues (Langeland *et al.*, 2006). Super and colleagues (2015) propose that empowerment and reflection enhance health promotion activities aiming to strengthen sense of coherence.

Engagement is also good for our health. Absorption in pursuits and activities beyond oneself are central to proposals for a psychology of positive emotions, aimed at understanding and building on our virtues and strengths (Seligman *et al.*, 2005; Ryff, 2014).

An English longitudinal study of almost 8,000 older people evaluated the relationship between happiness (positive affect), autonomy and purposeful engagement with life (*eudaemonia*) and various biological markers (Steptoe *et al.*, 2012). They found that both positive affect and eudaemonic well-being were associated with lower waist size in men, lower concentrations of inflammatory markers in women and with lower triglyceride levels and higher lung function in both genders. In studies conducted in the United States, older women with purposeful engagement and positive ties to others had lower plasma levels of inflammatory factors linked to a range of chronic diseases (Friedman *et al.*, 2007); while a sense of purpose in life, along with personal growth and positive affect, reduced the likelihood that low income would lead to the development of diabetes in older women in Wisconsin (Tsenkova *et al.*, 2007).

Kent and colleagues (2015) propose that engagement in terms of goal-directed actions, reflecting an individual's values and common humanity with others, can be enhanced through training. Their feasibility studies indicate beneficial effects on people living with post-traumatic stress disorder, obesity or chronic pain.

Expanding the scope of this dual-component concept of the self from depression more widely, including to patients living with long term conditions, appears to be intrinsically valuable. It moves us away from passive, mechanistic perspectives of disease, and provides the basis for constructive, life-enhancing conversations between people like Ken, living with chronic illness, and their health care providers. Joanne Reeve develops these ideas further in the next chapter, when she discusses the concept of creative capacity.

Agency, persons and selves

But for now, we have to consider some possible complicating factors.

Once we take a few steps further, and enquire whether the concept of the coherent, engaged self might provide a basis for understanding all our encounters in primary health care, then we begin to run into problems. These problems relate to the assumptions that we are all persons with agency, with the capacity to lead our own lives. This is important in primary health care, for example when we see patients with dementia or brain injuries, or with psychotic disorders such as schizophrenia.

Agency

Let us start with the notion of agency, defined as the capacity to lead our own lives, to undertake purposeful goal-directed activity, the power to make our own choices and decisions and take intentional action in a given environment (Anscombe, 2000).

Self-management regimes are predicated on the assumption that the sick person is highly motivated, highly health literate, and, paradoxically, in quite good health (May *et al.*, 2009). But in practice, we often find our agency subjected to more or less important constraints.

Our agency may be affected to varying degrees by our health. A common cold leaves us all less capable of purposeful goal-directed activity. My own ability to take intentional action has been reduced by a head injury which leaves me fatigued after a few hours of mental or physical activity. Ken's preference for racing pigeons has been curtailed by his lung disease. But for some people, such as Stephen Hawking with advanced amyotrophic lateral sclerosis, agency in a physical sense is so limited as to be virtually non-existent. Hawking retains the power to make choices and decisions, but taking action is impossible without the benefit of mechanical aids and other people. And for someone living with dementia, experiencing an acutely distressing psychotic episode or coming to terms with a head injury following a road traffic accident, the power to make choices may become dissipated, fragmented and even illusory.

Our agency may also be limited by the structures within which we find ourselves. My ability to act as a citizen of Europe is affected by the result of the UK 2016 referendum vote. Ken's working life on the docks was ended by decisions of the Liverpool Docks and Harbour Board, which itself was responding to national political pressures, a shift from open cargo to containerisation and a UK economy facing more towards Europe than the Americas. More significantly, people living in highly adverse circumstances have their power and their choices severely constrained, sometimes to the point of non-existence: those experiencing severe and sustained sexual abuse or domestic violence; or the relentlessly undermining effects of extreme poverty; or the cultural and political annihilation facing, for example, Jews living in Germany under the Nazi government, or members of the Yazidi community living in Isis-held northern Iraq.

Persons and selves

So far I have used the terms 'person' and 'self' interchangeably. However, if we want to expand concepts of coherence and engagement into primary health care more generally, I think it now becomes necessary to distinguish between these two terms.

If we accept John Locke's definition of a person as 'a thinking intelligent being, that has reason and reflection, and can consider itself as itself, the same thinking thing, in different times and places, which it does by that consciousness which is inseparable from thinking' (Locke, 1689, 2.27.9); and John Harris' more recent statement that 'a person will be any being capable of valuing its own existence' (Harris, 1985, p. 18), then we have to acknowledge that not all human beings fit this description.

Infants lack object permanence and are incapable of considering themselves as the same thinking thing in different times and places. So are those with severe brain damage or advanced dementia, who have lost the capacity for conceptual thought. People with schizophrenia experience a profound disruption of the self as subject, and often lack a sense of volition or agency.

If all human beings are not persons in the sense that Locke and Harris describe, we have a problem. If I do not value, or am not capable of valuing, my own existence, then others (including my family doctor) may consider they have the right to assign a lower priority to my needs in comparison to people who do value their own existence, or even to decide that my existence is surplus to society's requirements. From this point it is not difficult to imagine a two tier health system, or the beginnings of the slippery eugenic slope towards a neo-Nazi version of 'life unworthy of life' (Lifton, 1986).

Kant (1785) argues that respect for persons is an inalienable duty, which seems to be a step forward. However he bases our worthiness of respect on the assumption that reason is an essence of humanity, on our ability to choose right from wrong and to act as autonomous agents. Since we have already seen that not all human beings are capable of rational decision-making or autonomous action, this may not be adequate for our purposes.

One way out of this dilemma may be to distinguish formally between the person and the self. Even if not all human beings are persons, if we are or have a self then our right to dignity and respect can derive simply from this.

But this leads us on to a further question: what might a self be?

Self: experience or essence?

I think it is plausible to draw a distinction between the *experience* and the *essence* of the self. It may be generally accepted that self-experience exists, that all human beings have some degree of inner conscious presence, a sense of 'being me', and that most of us can observe and describe these experiences or phenomena. More contentious, is whether the self has an essence, an ontological reality; and, if so, of what that might consist.

Experiential selves

A self as something that is the subject of experience is a reasonable place to start, and gives us a basis for understanding and defending the rights of human beings. But we need to define this experiential self carefully, in order to encompass the range of patients we are likely to encounter in primary health care.

Three contemporary philosophers have helpful things to say on this subject: Galen Strawson on *single mental things*; Tim Bayne on *intentional entity;* and Barry Dainton on the *phenomenal self.*

Galen Strawson is confident that selves exist as subjects of experience. His formal phenomenological definition of self is 'a subject of experience that is a single, persisting mental thing that is an agent that has a certain personality and is not the same thing as a human being considered as a whole' (Strawson, 2009). He distinguishes between ordinary forms of self-experience, which include all these attributes, and minimal forms of self-experience which can exist in the absence of persistence, agency and a certain personality. This leaves him with the subject of experience as 'a single mental thing'.

Strawson's formulation of the self as a single mental thing makes sense for our purposes, insofar as the notion of persistence may be problematic for people who have major personality changes following brain injury, and I have previously noted both physical and social limitations to our sense of agency. However it still leaves us with some difficulties. The idea of the self as a single thing may be hard to accept for people with psychotic experiences of disintegration; and the mental component may be reduced to the point of insignificance for people with dementia.

Tim Bayne is interested in the unity of consciousness, in what it is like for me to be me. He distinguishes between basic 'creature consciousness', which includes background and specific conscious states; subject unity, which may be diachronic (persistent across time) or synchronic (persistent across different experiences at the same time); representational unity, the extent to which the contents of consciousness are integrated; and phenomenal unity or co-consciousness, the extent to which disparate experiences have a conjoint experiential character. For phenomenal unity he gives the example of sitting in a Cuban café in Paris, listening to rhumba on the stereo while watching a bartender mix a mojito and a dog chase its tail on the pavement outside, making notes and enjoying the anticipation of a lengthy trip (Bayne, 2010, p. 5).

Bayne sees the self as an *intentional entity*, with streams of consciousness constructed around a single intentional object. The self is a virtual centre of 'phenomenal gravity', 'an object whose identity is given by the intentional structure of the phenomenal field'. We appropriate to ourselves those experiences we are aware of. We assume that the character at the centre of our current stream of consciousness is the same as the character we are in contact with through our autobiographical memory. In making that assumption, says Bayne, we are 'not merely *tracking* ourselves but *creating* them' (Bayne, 2010, pp. 289–94). We are the creators of our own narratives, our own stories.

This self is not necessarily embodied, which allows Bayne to extend his definition to people with experience of depersonalisation. His concept of intentional entity also links well with Spinoza's *conatus*, with our desire to persist in our being. But his definitions may have limitations for people with schizophrenia, for whom loss of unity of consciousness is a core feature, and for whom intention can be severely depleted.

More compelling, to me, is Barry Dainton's argument for a *phenomenal* self, based on continuity of consciousness (Dainton, 2008; 2014). He proposes that we are each a collection of persisting capacities for experience, and that the self is reducible to its experiences. The subject – the self – is something with the *continuous capacity* to be conscious. It has the ability to stream experiences over time, with a single uninterrupted potential for experience. Although our immediate experience occurs in the present, this phenomenal present is successively linked to others in a co-conscious stream, and there is continuity of the self if phases of consciousness overlap. We don't have to be conscious all the time – we are able to sleep dreamlessly – it is sufficient that we have the *capacity* to be conscious.

Dainton's self exists within a phenomenal world, although the phenomena it experiences may be virtual, as in advanced computer gaming technology and teleportation. He gives (currently) hypothetical examples from advanced gaming, in which I might become – for a predetermined period of time – a historical character such as Napoleon at the Battle of Waterloo or a U-Boat commander on patrol in the Atlantic. Although I lose psychological continuity, in that I perceive myself to be Napoleon or the U-Boat commander, I continue to exist insofar as my consciousness continues to flow without interruption.

What is valuable here is that advanced virtual reality gaming suggests that the self can survive psychological rupture. Dainton's concept of the self does not depend on biographical memory or psychological continuity, but simply on the capacity to stream experiences. It is therefore consistent with what we understand of dementia (when biographical memory may be lost) and of brain injury (where psychological continuity may be absent).

So, how does all this help me to understand my patient Harry, who is living with dementia?

Harry is 85 and a retired head teacher. He's recently been admitted to a local care home, as his family found it impossible to keep him safe in his own home, and subsequently in sheltered accommodation. His main problem is moderately severe Alzheimer's disease, with scores of 21/28 on the six item cognitive impairment test and 4/10 on the abbreviated mental test score.

His social skills are in good working order, but he appears to have reverted to life as a headmaster. He gets irritated with the staff when they do not follow his instructions. Harry is convinced that he is due to retire, so keeps on packing all his belongings away so that the next head teacher can take over his room.

He has also been politely apprehended while trying to make his escape with a ladder over the back garden wall.

According to the perspectives presented in this section, Harry's sense of self remains firmly intact. He experiences himself as a single mental thing with persistence (I do not have to agree with him about exactly what form that persistence takes) and the care staff certainly see him as an agent with a personality. He is an intentional entity, crafting his own narratives, recreating his misplaced world of school-mastery. And, although his biographical memory is severely disrupted, he retains the capacity to stream his experiences over time.

Essential selves

The next question to consider is whether our phenomenological experience of the self, or sense of 'being me', is based on any specific reality; in philosophical terms, whether the self has an essence, an ontological or metaphysical reality.

In this section I consider four different contemporary philosophical positions for an understanding of the essential self: *embodied self; social and distributed self; no-self; and multiple selves.* I provide a summary of each position and suggest how it links into the elements of personhood or selfhood which I have previously discussed.

Embodied self

Anil Ananthaswamy (2015) proposes a minimal self, capable of being the subject of an experience at any given moment: a pre-cognitive, pre-reflective self, necessarily embedded in the body. Like Stefán Hjörleifsson and Kjersti Lea in Chapter 2, he draws on Merleau-Ponty (1958) to support the idea that our bodily habits, gestures and actions convey our humanness and individuality He also brings in Bourdieu's *habitus* (1977), where the body incorporates our social and cultural customs. For people living with schizophrenia, he sees a minimal self, distinct from the extended narrative self, whose sense of agency may be reduced by the lack of predictability but who remains the subject that is experiencing psychosis. Ananthaswamy agrees with Dainton that the self does not depend on narrative, and is separate and independent from cognition.

Social and distributed self

Tom Kitwood and Kathleen Bredin (1992) propose that personhood (though I would restate this as 'selfhood' for reasons noted above) 'should be viewed as essentially social: it refers to the human being in relation to others'. In the same way that the transformation of a neonate into a being who has the full range of human attributes is a social process, and not one of simple maturation, the fragmentary effects of dementia may be mitigated through human interaction, rather than a process of inevitable degeneration. They envisage a continuum of selfhood from *shattered* (as in psychosis or dementia) through *frozen* (as in unsupported everyday competence) to *fluid* (as in fully relational) and see interdependence as a necessary condition of being human: 'A more desirable form of life would be one in which there was vastly more intersubjectivity, and where there would be a continuing opportunity for people to be fluid; or, to alter the image, to grow and change' (Kitwood and Brewin, 1992).

So for Harry, the extent and speed at which his mental functioning deteriorates, and any consequent suffering he may experience, will be mediated by his relationships with his family, his friends and the staff in his residential home. And there remains the possibility that it will not simply be a case of slowing deterioration, but that his social interactions may enable changes which – even if he cannot communicate them to others – may represent something new and positive for his sense of self, his being.

Harry has recently joined a reading group and contributes to the discussions in a very cogent and deep way. When the group were reading John Keats' poem '*A thing of beauty if a joy for ever*', Harry spoke about it being a good life philosophy to have, but one that can be difficult to get into 'if you are on the outside of it.' And, when listening to a reading from Mary Shelley's Frankenstein, he wondered what it would be like to be 'rejected, to be rejected'.

It may be that these relational experiences are helping Harry give shape to the profound changes in his own selfhood.

This links with Martin Buber's *Ich-Du* (I-Thou) relationship, the mutual holistic exchange of two beings who meet without qualification or objectification of the other. Working on the premise of existence as encounter, Buber gives examples as diverse as two lovers, an observer and a cat, the author and a tree, and two strangers on a train, to show how my own self appears and grows as I recognise the other (Buber, 2008); a valuable insight for primary care professionals to reflect on, during encounters with our patients. This also provides a basis for the notion of 'shared mind' in the consultation, to which I will return later in this chapter.

The *distributed* self includes the social self but also – critically – involves non-human agents. Sherry Turkle (2005) sees individuals as an amalgamation of distinct selves, distributed across space (and time) and including computers. Stephen Hawking would be completely unable to function, to express his self, without the benefit of highly sophisticated technology, and we can reasonably assume that his self has been adapted as a result of these incessant, essential interactions. In combination with the otherwise inert machines he is attached to, he continues to provide startling insights into the mysteries of the universe.

No self

Perhaps there is no essential self at all. In Buddhist philosophy, *Anattā (*no-self) is, along with *Dukkha* (suffering) and *Anicca* (impermanence), one of the three 'right understandings' about existence. In Buddhism it is important for me to become increasingly self-aware, to attend to my own psychological state through meditation, while paradoxically loosening my relationship with and my attachment to my idea of the self (Lesser, 2013). The first person presentation in the content of consciousness, the sense of ownership of mineness, of 'being me', is ultimately an error, an illusion, a fiction (Ganeri, 2012).

For philosopher Julian Baggini, the self is a psychological delusion, a systematic misconception of agency; 'the ego trick is to create something which has a strong sense of unity and singleness from what is actually a messy, fragmented sequence of experiences and memories' (Baggini, 2011). The experimental psychologist Bruce Hood also sees the self as an illusion. In reality, he argues, we are composed of a multitude of competing urges and impulses. Developmental processes shape our brains from infancy onwards to create our identities, while systematic biases distort the content of our identity to form a consistent narrative (Hood, 2012).

A common element in these arguments is against psychological continuity as a valid basis for a self. But if we acknowledge that psychological ruptures can occur – as in schizophrenia, traumatic brain injuries, or advanced dementia – and follow Dainton in arguing that these are not of fundamental importance to our identity or existence, then we do not have to abandon the notion of a continuous conscious self. And, as Cees van Leeuwen argues, cognitive neuroscience may be biased in favour of assuming an illusory experience of unity because of its own emphasis on functional specialisation and localisation. He suggests, as an equally plausible hypothesis, that our experience of unity is afforded by the intrinsic, adaptive multi-scale dynamics of the brain (van Leeuwen, 2015).

Multiple selves

Galen Strawson (2009) acknowledges minimal forms of genuine self-experience, which can exist in the absence of persistence, agency and personality. But he is not convinced that a continuous self actually exists. In contrast to Dainton, he argues that a subject of experience can only exist if experience exists of which it is the subject. Gaps in experience (during periods of dreamless sleep, for example) mean that there are also gaps in the subject. The subject must be live, in order to exist at all.

He argues towards the concept of *thin* selves, which may be many, short-lived and transient. He combines analytical philosophy with Buddhism (and many other elements) to propose that, while we may consider ourselves to be single subjects of experience, this coherence dissolves in the face of our inner mental subjectivity:

> I feel I have continuity through the waking day only as an embodied human being.... When I consider myself in the whole-human-being way I fully endorse the conventional view that there is in my case – that I am – a single subject of experience – a person – with long-term diachronic continuity. But when I experience myself as an inner mental subject and consider the detailed character of conscious experience, my feeling is that I am – that the thing that I most essentially am is – continually completely new.
>
> (Strawson, 2009, p. 247)

For me, Strawson's multiple selves, his sense of being continually and completely new, are exciting and liberating. Ken, Harry and I are not necessarily and irretrievably trapped within any particular way of viewing the world or our own positions within it. My self is neither fixed nor determined. I exist – with the perpetual potential to change, to grow, to flourish. Perhaps one day, like Raimund Gregorius, I will board the night train for Lisbon (Mercier, 2008) and discover an entirely different version of the many lives I could have lived. Or perhaps I will continue to live the life I have, but enjoy it ever more fully and intensely.

Conclusions

Coherent engaged self

These perspectives, despite their differences, offer us the possibility of retaining the concept of a coherent and engaged self, now in a stripped-down, elemental form.

While not all human beings are persons in the formal sense proposed by Locke and Harris, have innate rationality as understood by Kant, or retain sufficient agency to allow them to lead their own lives in ways that matter to them, the propositions discussed in this chapter permit the formulation of a concept of the self which is worthy of dignity and respect in its own right.

Reflecting on *coherence* and its four original elements, I may have to relinquish the element of curiosity, in relation to the negative symptoms of schizophrenia, and the element of memory in relation to dementia. I am reassured that this loss may not be too serious by Stephen Katz' persuasive argument for the normalcy and indeed necessity of forgetting, as a liberating antidote to the 'relentless horizons of experience' (Katz, 2012). But the element of imagination has not been seriously questioned, and I submit that the element of desire or endeavour (probably the most important of all) is still broadly intact. We saw earlier in the chapter how Spinoza, in his definition of *conatus*, specifically refers to the desire of mind 'both in so far as it has clear and distinct ideas and in so far as it has confused ideas', which allows for its persistence across altered mental states and is not dependent on psychological continuity; and (with the caveats noted earlier) is consistent with Bayne's intentional entity.

If I am formulating coherence on the basis of self-experience, then I am on reasonably comfortable ground with Dainton's phenomenal self, based on continuity of consciousness. But the argument does become more complicated if I am aiming to establish an essential self as the basis for coherence, given the heterogeneity of conceptual possibilities.

The concept of the embodied minimal self is plausible for human beings with reduced capacity, such as those with severe traumatic brain injury or Alzheimer's disease, and is consistent with the call within contemporary dementia scholarship for the deconstruction of 'cerebral selfhood' and a greater reliance on subtle bodily signs of distress and discomfort, of joy and pleasure (Downs, 2013).

Importantly, the embodied self also works well for human beings more generally, in states of heightened physical awareness, such as sexual arousal and orgasm, mountain climbing, running or cycling uphill. I have written previously about the sense of 'being alive' that comes from intense physical activity, in this case a recent cycle ride in the wind and rain when I ended up with numb feet, drenched right through to the skin.

> There is something fundamentally important about being fully in the moment, in touch with my body and with the world around me, engaging all my senses. It's about immediate, direct, physical, sensuous reality. Undoubtable existence. It's about now. Whatever happens later doesn't matter.
>
> (Dowrick, 2012)

Thought is at a minimum. All my usual mental chatter and self-judgement disappear. I am my body.

The Buddhist no-self is problematic for proponents of an essential self, though paradoxically it is strongly linked with heightened self-awareness, and cognitive neuroscience is in flux on the subject. While recommending the concept of multiple thin selves, Strawson acknowledges that these selves are coherent entities in their own right. He believes Spinoza to be fundamentally correct in asserting the reality of human subjectivity within the one subject of experience, the universe: 'it is true that there is diversity but also true that it is, somehow, all one' (Strawson, 2009, p. 424).

My concept of the self assumes our *engagement* with the world. The evidence presented in this chapter, especially the section on the social self, does nothing to negate this assumption, though it does indicate the need for some modifications. Implicit in my original version was a sense of *active* engagement, of our positively choosing to be involved in moral practices or with the routines of everyday life. I think this now needs to be extended to include reactive or *receptive* elements of engagement, including being cared for by other people, or gaining benefit from encounters with machines and technology. Engagement necessitates the social, even when (as at the beginning and the end of life, or if we are living with disability) this takes forms of engaging with others to have our own basic needs met.

Conceptual implications

To return to my opening statement in this chapter, I consider that we need a concept of the self which provides all patients with dignity and respect during their encounters in primary health care, and offers a basis for receiving equitable treatment according to their needs.

The original version of my concept of the coherent and engaged self does offer all this but, as I have indicated, may not be applicable to the lives and experiences of every patient seeking help from primary care practitioners. So my proposition now is as follows:

> the concept of the coherent and engaged self, with coherence based on the capacity to be continuously conscious, and engagement including receptive as well as active elements, is widely applicable and provides an ethical foundation for patient-centred care.

Given my concerns about the definitions of the word 'person', I am not convinced that 'person-centred care' is an entirely reliable term, even though it is the title of this book. Although I would argue that 'self-centred care' is more accurate, the ambiguities of that term are so complex that I think 'patient-centred care' is the safest option.

Of course, while the ability to establish arguments for a minimal patient self may be a necessary precondition of ensuring an equitable and ethical health care system, it should not be assumed that concern for one's self is the primary aim of human existence. At the level of political philosophy, we find Millbank and Pabst (2016) arguing for a civil economy within which the rights of the individual are blended with principles of reciprocity and mutuality. And in Buddhist philosophy, no-self (*anattā*), arises out of concern for the suffering of others (Ganeri, 2012). Attachment to the self is a kind of dysfunction, and losing that attachment is liberation.

Implications for practice

For primary health care professionals, understanding and recognising the other, the patient, as a self with intrinsic worth, offers liberation from restricted and restricting attachments to our medical world views and reduces the risk of doctor-centred encounters in the consultation. It encourages us to engage with the selves of our patients, with skill, curiosity and wonder.

The concept of the coherent and engaged self also provides the foundation for a range of perspectives which have in common the presumption of a substantial patient voice. Three of these perspectives are particularly noteworthy: *shared mind*; *allocating the work of disease*; and the *proactive work of patient-hood.*

Shared mind

While the coherent self provides a rationale for seeing the patient as a worthy entity in their own right, the engaged self, with its social or distributed elements, brings to the fore the importance of the relationship between patient and practitioner. Ronald Epstein advocates the notion of shared mind, the ways in which new ideas and perspectives can emerge through sharing thoughts, feelings, perceptions, meanings, and intentions among two or more people (Epstein and Street, 2011; Epstein, 2013). Grounded in assumptions that autonomy and decision-making are not the exclusive preserve of the professional, shared mind not only builds on but also enhances these attributes in the patient.

Ken comes to see me for one of his regular medication reviews. After I've listened to his chest and checked his peak flow, I ask him how his health is affecting his life. He is pleased with himself for stopping smoking but expresses concern that I will disapprove of his whisky chasers and betting on the horses.

I start to explain the impact of alcohol on his gastritis and the effects of betting-related stress on his breathing, but then, in mid-sentence, I stop.

We look at each other, start to smile and then end up laughing: at my pomposity, at the medically-focussed absurdity of our conversation. 'I'm sorry Ken', I say, 'I guess that's all a bit trivial in the grand scheme of things.' Ken agrees. 'I know I haven't got that long left, Prof., but what the hell, I do need some fun in my life.'

What does it matter if Ken drinks a bit more than the latest health guidance tells us he should? The meanings of his life, rooted in his family and his experiences on the docks, are not in any way affected by how many years more or less he ends up living. Our shared mind is clear: Ken can and should choose how he spends the time remaining to him.

Meanwhile, retired headmaster Harry has made another bid for freedom from his residential home.

Harry's carers worry about their ability to keep him safe, and raise the question of sedative medication.

Harry and I sit together in his room to discuss what has been happening, and what we should do. I discover that the attempts to leave the premises usually occur late afternoon, and, for Harry, the problem is clear: 'It's the end of the school day and I want to get off home, but these folks are just getting in my way and stopping me. Really, they have no right to do so.'

I agree with him that must be very frustrating, and offer to have a word with the staff. They agree to take him out for a walk in the afternoon, around school closing time. That seems to make a big difference to Harry, who is much more relaxed as a result.

Even though Harry and I do not have the same analysis of the problems he is experiencing, we do have shared mind in that we can exchange thoughts and feelings and, with the help of the staff in the care home, construct some commonly agreed meanings and intentions which lead to mutually beneficial actions.

Shared mind may also be used by practitioners in protective ways. One example would be when a patient is in the depths of despair but, nevertheless, retains a degree of confidence in the therapeutic relationship. On several such occasions I have promised a patient that I will 'hold on to your hope for you, until you are ready to take it back again'. I have subsequently been assured that this offer, even if the possibility was not fully believed at the time, was much appreciated.

Allocating the work of disease

These concepts also offer an entry point for understanding how the work of disease is allocated, the ways in which doctors and patients come together to enact illness, the common object of their concerns. As Annemarie Mol explored the work involved with atherosclerosis in the lower limbs, she found patients to be far more than passive victims of disease or inactive recipients of care. They were actively engaged. When she asked the crucial question 'Who does the doing?' she found doctor and patient on a par. Each had multiple roles to perform, though these roles were fluid and their scripts were not predetermined. 'When doctor and patient act together in the consulting room, they jointly give shape to the reality of the patient's hurting leg'. The performance of disease requires coordination and distribution of activities amongst all concerned. There is mutual inclusion. As with Buber, 'to be is to be related'. And we find that it is not only minds that are shared. 'Day to day reality, the life we live, is also a fleshy affair' (Mol, 2002, p. 27).

Ultimately, it is patients who make normative decisions: these may be on the basis of the market, as customer buying wares; or on the basis of their position as citizens, seeing medicine as a set of interventions into modes of living, over which they, crucially, have jurisdiction.

Proactive work of patient-hood

The coherent, engaged self also provides vital underpinning for the new proactive work of patient-hood, for which patients are increasingly accountable. Ideas about self-care, self-empowerment, and self-actualisation are becoming prominent, and new technologies and treatment modalities are being shifted from the clinic into the community. As Carl May has demonstrated (May *et al.*, 2014), these apparently benign ideological and organisational changes place new demands on sick people, which they may experience as burdens of treatment.

In response, as we have seen, patients like Ken and Harry have agency. They can do things to engage with their health problems and with other people. They can mobilise capacity, build up their potential to absorb adversity and capitalise on their informational and material resources. 'Patients and their relational networks can act as collective agents to invest in work' needed to address their health problems, though agency and work are 'unstable situational accomplishments' which have to be continually reproduced (May *et al.*, 2014).

For Ken and Harry, I am a part of their relational networks. I have the opportunity, indeed the responsibility, to work together with them to make the most of their agency, to enable them to make their lives as comfortable, as full of meaning, as possible.

Key learning points

1   In relation to depression, a concept of the coherent, engaged self, of persons with the capacity to lead their lives, provides a basis for a strong understanding of the patient self.
2   This concept has wider applicability, including for people living with long term conditions.
3   It is more useful than the passive, mechanistic views of the patient commonly adopted by doctors steeped in the physical sciences.
4   However it needs refining in relation to people with reduced capacity, including acknowledging a distinction between persons and selves.
5   Self-experience, based on capacity for continuity of consciousness, is a candidate to be the basis of coherence.
6   Self-essence might be embodied, social, non-existent or continually renewed.
7   The engaged self may be receptive as well as active, involving technology as well as other people.

8   The coherent and engaged self, in minimal form, provides an ethical basis for respect for patients.

9   The coherent and engaged self also offers a foundation for mutual encounters between patients and health professionals, encouraging shared mind and enabling patients to work with their illnesses.

References

Ananthaswamy, A. 2015. *The man who wasn't there.* New York: Dutton.

Anscombe, E. 2000. *Intention.* Cambridge: Harvard University Press.

Antonovsky, A. 1987. Unravelling the mystery of health: how people manage stress and stay well. San Francisco: Jossey-Bass, p. 18.

Baggini, J. 2011. *The ego trick.* London: Granta.

Bayne, T. 2010. *The unity of consciousness.* Oxford: Oxford University Press.

Boeckxstaens, P., Vaes, B., De Sutter, A., Aujoulat, I., van Pottelbergh, G., Matheï, C., Degryse, J.M. 2016. A high sense of coherence as protection against adverse health outcomes in patients aged 80 years and older. *Annals of Family Medicine,* 14 (4): 337–43.

Bourdieu, P. 1977. *Outline of a theory of practice.* Cambridge: Cambridge University Press.

Buber, M. 2008. *Ich und du.* Stuttgart: Reclam.

Camus, A. 1942. *Le mythe de Sisyphe.* Paris: Gallimard.

Craig, A. 2009. How do you feel – now? *Nature Reviews Neuroscience,* 10 (1): 59–70.

Dainton, B. 2008. *The phenomenal self.* Oxford: Oxford University Press.

Dainton, B. 2014. *Self.* London: Penguin.

Downs, M. 2013. Embodiment. *Dementia,* 12 (3): 368–74.

Dowrick, C. 2009. *Beyond depression,* 2nd edition. Oxford: Oxford University Press.

Dowrick, C. 2012. *Feeling alive.* Wellbecoming blog. Available at: http://wellbecoming. blogspot.co.uk/2012/05/feeling-alive.html (accessed 8 May 2017).

Dowrick, C. 2016. Suffering, Meaning and Hope. *In:* Wakefield, J., Demazeux, S. (eds) *Sadness or depression?* New York: Springer, pp. 121–36.

Epstein, R.M. 2013. Whole mind and shared mind in clinical decision-making. *Patient Education and Counselling,* 90 (2): 200–6.

Epstein, R.M. and Street, R.L. Jr. 2011. Shared mind. *Annals of Family Medicine,* 9 (5): 454–61.

Farrelly, S., Lester, H., Rose, D., Birchwood, M., Marshall, M., Waheed, W., Henderson, R.C., Szmukler, G. and Thornicroft, G. 2015. Improving therapeutic relationships. *Qualitative Health Research,* 25 (12): 1637–47.

Fernros, L., Furhoff, A.K. and Wändell. P.E. 2008. Improving quality of life using compound mind-body therapies: evaluation of a course intervention with body movement and breath therapy, guided imagery, chakra experiencing and mindfulness meditation. *Quality of Life Research,* 17: 367–76.

Friedman, E.M., Hayney, M., Love, G.D., Singer, B.H. and Ryff, C.D. 2007. Plasma interleukin-6 and soluble IL-6 receptors are associated with psychological well-being in aging women. *Health Psychology,* 26 (3): 305–13.

Ganeri, J. 2012. *The self.* Oxford: Oxford University Press.

Griffiths, F.E., Boardman, F.K., Chondros, P., Dowrick, C.F., Densley, K., Hegarty, K.L. and Gunn, J. 2015. The effect of strategies of personal resilience on depression recovery in an Australian cohort: a mixed methods study. *Health,* 19 (1): 86–106.

Harris, J. 1985. *The value of life.* London: Routledge.

Heidegger, M. 1996. *Being and time* (Stambaugh, J., trans.). Albany: University of New York.

Hood, B. 2012. *The self illusion.* London: Constable and Robinson.

Kant, I. 1785. *Fundamental principles of the metaphysic of morals* (10th ed.). Abbott, T.K., ed. Project Gutenberg.

Katz, S. 2012. Embodied memory. *Occasion: Interdisciplinary Studies in the Humanities,* 4 (May 31). Available at: http://occasion.stanford.edu/node/97

Keil, D.C., Vaske, I., Kenn, K., Rief, W. and Stenzel, N.M. 2017. With the strength to carry on. *Chronic Respiratory Disease,* 14 (1): 11–21.

Kent, M., Rivers, C.T. and Wrenn, G. 2015. Goal-Directed Resilience in Training (GRIT). *Behavioral Science,* 5 (2): 264–304.

Kitwood, T. and Bredin, K. 1992. Towards a theory of dementia care. *Ageing and Society,* 12: 269–87.

Kontos, P. and Martin, W. 2013. Embodiment and dementia. *Dementia,* 12(3): 288–302.

Langeland, E., Riise, T., Hanestad, B.R., Nortvedt, M.W., Kristoffersen, K. and Wahl, A.K. 2006. The effect of salutogenic treatment principles on coping with mental health problems: a randomised controlled trial. *Patient Education and Counselling,* 62 (2): 212–19.

Lehtinen, V., Sohlman, B., Nummelin, T., Salomaa, M., Ayuso-Mateos, J.L. and Dowrick, C. 2005. The estimated incidence of depressive disorder and its determinants in the Finnish ODIN sample. *Social Psychiatry and Psychiatric Epidemiology,* 40: 778–84.

Lesser, M. 2013. *Know yourself forget yourself.* Novato: New World Library.

Lifton, R.J. 1986. *The Nazi doctors.* New York: Basic Books.

Locke, J. 1689. *Essays concerning human understanding.* Oxford: Oxford University Press.

Lynch, J., Moore, M., Moss-Morris, R. and Kendrick, T. 2015. Do patients' illness beliefs predict depression measures at six months in primary care? *Journal of Affective Disorders,* 174: 665–71.

MacIntyre, A. (1984) *After virtue: a study in moral theory,* 2nd edition. Notre Dame Indiana: University of Notre Dame Press.

Martel. Y. 2002. *Life of Pi: a novel.* Edinburgh: Canongate.

May, C.R., Montori, V.M. and Mair, F.S. 2009. We need minimally disruptive medicine. *British Medical Journal,* 339: b2803.

May, C.R., Eton, D.T., Boehmer, K., Gallacher, K., Hunt, K., MacDonald, S., Mair, F.S., May, C.M., Montori, V.M., Richardson, A., Rogers, A.E. and Shippee, N. 2014. Rethinking the patient: using Burden of Treatment Theory to understand the changing dynamics of illness. *BMC Health Services Research,* 14: 281.

Mercier, P. 2008. *Night train to Lisbon* (Harshaw, B., trans.). London: Atlantic Books.

Millbank, J. and Pabst, A. 2016. *The politics of virtue.* Lanham: Rowman and Littlefield.

Merleau-Ponty, M. 1958. *Les sciences de l'homme et la phenomenologie.* Paris: Centre de Documentation Universitaire.

Mol, A.M. 2002. *The body multiple.* Durham: Duke University Press.

Nilsen, V., Bakke, P.S., Rohde, G. and Gallefoss, F. 2015. Is sense of coherence a predictor of lifestyle changes in subjects at risk for type 2 diabetes? *Public Health,* 129 (2): 155–61.

Proust, M. 2002. *In search of lost time. Volume 1: Swann's way* (Scott Moncrieff C.K., Kilmartin, T. and Enright, D.J., trans.). London: Vintage Press, pp. 51–5.

Pusswald, G., Fleck, M., Lehrner, J., Haubenberger, D., Weber, G. and Auff, E. 2012. The 'Sense of Coherence' and the coping capacity of patients with Parkinson disease. *International Psychogeriatrics*, 24 (12): 1972–9.

Ross, W.D. 1953. *Aristotle's Metaphysics*. Oxford: Clarendon Press.

Ryff, C.D. 2014. Psychological well-being revisited. *Psychotherapy and Psychosomatics*, 83 (1): 10–28.

Seligman, M.E., Steen, T.A., Park, N. and Peterson, C. 2005. Positive psychology progress: empirical validation of interventions. *American Psychology*, 60: 410–21

Simpson, J. 1997. *Touching the void*. New York: Vintage.

Skelton, J.R., Wearn, A.M. and Hobbs, F.D. 2002. A concordance-based study of metaphoric expressions used by general practitioners and patients in consultation. *British Journal of General Practice*, 52 (475): 114–18.

Spinoza, B. 2000. *Ethics* (Parkinson, G.H.R., ed. and trans.). Oxford: Oxford University Press.

Steptoe, A., Demakakos, P., de Oliveira, C. and Wardle, J. 2012. Distinctive biological correlates of positive psychological well-being in older men and women. *Psychosomatic Medicine*, 74 (5): 501–8.

Strawson, G. 2009. *Selves*. Oxford: Oxford University Press.

Super, S., Verschuren, W.M., Zantinge, E.M., Wagemakers, M.A. and Picavet, H.S. 2014. A weak sense of coherence is associated with a higher mortality risk. *Journal of Epidemiology and Community Health*, 68 (5): 411–17.

Super, S., Wagemakers, M.A., Picavet, H.S., Verkooijen, K.T. and Koelen, M.A. 2015. Strengthening sense of coherence. *Health Promotion International*, July 23, p. ii.

Taylor, C. 1989. *Sources of the self: the making of the modern identity*. Cambridge: Cambridge University Press.

Tsenkova, V.K., Love, G.D., Singer, B.H. and Ryff, C.D. 2007. Socioeconomic status and psychological well-being predict cross-time change in glycosylated hemoglobin in older women without diabetes. *Psychosomatic Medicine*, 69: 777–84.

Turkle, S. 2005. *The second self*. Cambridge: MIT Press.

van Leeuwen, C. 2015. What makes you think you are conscious? *Frontiers of Human Neuroscience*, 9: 170.

Vogel, I., Miksch, A., Goetz, K., Ose, D., Szecsenyi, J. and Freund, T. 2012. The impact of perceived social support and sense of coherence on health-related quality of life in multimorbid primary care patients. *Chronic Illness*, 8 (4): 296–307.

Wainwright, N.W., Surtees, P.G., Welch, A.A., Luben, R.N., Khaw, K.T. and Bingham, S.A. 2008. Sense of coherence, lifestyle choices and mortality. *Journal of Epidemiology and Community Health*, 62 (2): 829–31.

Wiesmann, U., Dezutter, J. and Hannich, H.J. 2014. Sense of coherence and pain experience in older age. *International Psychogeriatrics*, 26 (1): 123–33.

Wollheim, R. 1984. *The thread of life*. Cambridge: Cambridge University Press.

Zeldin, T. 1994. *An intimate history of humanity*. London: Sinclair-Stevenson.

7   Unlocking the creative capacity of the self

Joanne Reeve

General practice: dealing with the ill person

It is gone 6 pm when I call in my last patient. It has been a long day – I started at 7.30 am and will have another hour of paperwork to complete when I have seen this person. Heather has been added on the end of my list as an urgent patient having arrived at reception and asked to see a doctor straightaway. It just says 'very unwell' on my list. Heather walks through the door helped by her friend, sits down, whispers 'I feel so ill', and dissolves into tears. I mentally put my pile of paperwork to one side, and turn my full attention on the person sat in front of me.

I am a General Practitioner (GP). My job is to manage whoever and whatever walks through my door. In many ways, Heather's story is typical. People come to see me because they feel ill – something is upsetting their experience of day to day living, and they believe (worry) that the disturbance is health-related. They come and seek advice and help from a doctor – someone who can help them understand what is happening and so help them deal with the problem. If asked, many would perhaps describe a hope that the doctor will be able to 'make it better' – tell them how to solve the problem. But most also know that it may not be that straightforward.

As a GP, my job is therefore to deal with illness – health needs that are defined by the individual patients that I see. Yet most of my early medical training was focused on disease – identifying and managing deviation from anatomical, physiological or biochemical norms. In my medical training, health needs were defined by professionals and health systems. Even within my formal GP training, the focus on illness has been limited.

This gap is what led me into the world of research. I wanted to understand more about illness, and how to offer illness-focused care. Illness is a personal experience and I soon discovered that to understand illness, I had to also explore and understand who was the person – or more appropriately, the self (as Christopher Dowrick argued in the previous chapter) – who came into my consulting room. So I embarked on an exploration of what it is to be ill, specifically work to understand the self who is living with illness. My goal is to consider how I as a physician can work with individuals to support them in dealing with their illness.

Introducing the Creative Self

My understanding of the ill self has evolved over a yet unfinished lifetime of professional practice – stimulated by my contact with patients, expanded through reflections on the writing of some great scholars, and developed further through my own research. I started my exploration with a mental image of the ill person caught adrift in the ever-flowing river of daily life. Something deep – an innate sense of survival, an 'inner self' – keeps them afloat and looking to navigate to safer ground. Calm waters may allow the ill self to drift a while, even paddle gently. But if the flow of life becomes more turbulent – perhaps in response to the illness – that survival becomes harder. Our ill person may be cast adrift with only a flimsy piece of driftwood to cling to as they are rocked by the waves; others may have the added stability of a canoe. Whether they are treading water (perhaps whilst waiting for rescue), or moving onward to safety, the ill person is working to navigate the flow of daily life. Ideally they have access to oars to help power through the waves; although some may only have their hands and feet to paddle with. Some individuals find themselves with both canoe and oars, yet still struggle to sail through the rocky waves. For these ill selves, the problem may lie in what is loaded within the boat. Heavy loads may slow progress but still allow forward momentum. More disruptive is an imbalanced load which may, faced with a turbulent flow, cause the individual to be diverted off course (Figure 7.1).

In this chapter, I will describe how I have developed these thoughts into a concept of the Creative Self – an account of the self which focuses on the response of an individual to the ups and downs of daily living. I understand health as a necessary resource for daily living (Williamson and Carr, 2009); being part of agency – the innate capacity or potential of all human beings to live their own life, changing and progressing in recognition of and response to both internal and external stimuli (Dowrick, 2004; Carel, 2008; Reeve and Cooper, 2016). The account that I will develop and describe reveals the enactment of this self-agency to be dependent on the interplay of five elements which influence the successful mobilisation of the 'creative capacity' of the self (Carel, 2008) in response to illness. My account of the Creative Self proposes that faced with illness, the goal for both the individual and the professional working with them

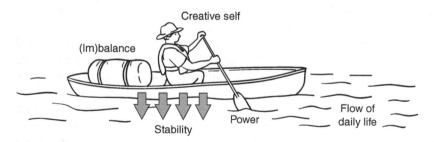

Figure 7.1 Imagining the Creative Self.

is to realise the capacity of the Creative Self – to support individual self-agency in restoring daily living.

I start this chapter by describing the development of my account of the Creative Self. I then consider how I am using this work to help clinicians to better understand their role in managing the ill self, whilst also prompting redesign of services to better deliver self-focused care at scale.

Exploring illness and discovering the self

My earliest professional experiences of dealing with the gap between the needs of the ill self and the priorities of clinical medicine nearly took me out of medicine and off down a different career path. Instead, I found myself starting a PhD – an opportunity to explore in depth the overlap and dissonance between biomedical and personal interpretations of illness. I opted to look specifically at the illness experience recognised as depressed mood and for both theoretical and pragmatic reasons, the patient group I chose were those living with advanced terminal cancer.

Biomedical teaching at the time encouraged us to screen individuals with terminal cancer for depression. Evidence suggested that the use of antidepressants even in the final weeks of life could improve depression scores. My project set out to explore how depression score ratings of 'depression' related to individual's own perceptions of their health needs.

I began the work anticipating I would see some overlap and some disagreement between the two perspectives. What I didn't expect was that in a collection of 19 in-depth interviews, conducted using an interview schedule designed to explore experiences of depressed mood, I found very little data on depression. Instead, I found rich accounts of people's efforts to live their daily lives – adapting where they needed to, and where they could, to the effects of cancer, terminal illness, health services and distress. People talked about their mood, but it was a relatively small part of a much larger conversation – even in those who, biomedically speaking, scored as having moderate-severe depression. These accounts took my thesis off in a completely different direction.

In seeking to make sense of these stories of illness, I turned to the sociological literature describing the impact of illness on biography – peoples' stories of daily living. In the early 1980s, Bury (1982) first outlined an account of chronic illness as biographical disruption. He proposed that illness upsets the structures of daily life and the knowledge that underpins them, creating new work for the individual above and beyond the direct effects of the illness itself. Subsequent research was to challenge Bury's original description, arguing that his account of 'fractured' narratives was overstated with new findings instead highlighting the adaptive response of individuals supporting a continuity of narrative, albeit with change (Williams, 1984, 2000; Faircloth et al., 2004). This literature was to help move my thinking from a focus on distress, to looking at adaptation and agency; work which coincided with, and was supported by, Dowrick's (2004) publication of *Beyond Depression*. But which also generated many questions about how people could respond and adapt. I wanted to understand what individuals were doing, what helped and hindered in this process, and with what implications for my role as a generalist physician.

It was around this time that I discovered Havi Carel – a philosopher whose work considers what it is to be ill, based on a scholarly exploration of her own experiences of an unexpected diagnosis of a life-limiting illness. Carel's (2008) writing helped open up my interpretation of the stories being told to me by my research participants, and in turn my understanding of the relationship between illness and the self.

Having been previously fit and well, in her thirties Carel started to experience breathing problems – extreme breathlessness associated with even minor activity. As her symptoms worsened, she sought medical help. She was diagnosed with a rare, progressive, and ultimately fatal disease – lymphangioleiomyomatosis. This episode was certainly disruptive to her daily living, and prompted her as a philosopher to look at how we describe and discuss illness. Carel describes her early experience of illness as being characterised by the 'betrayal of [her] body' (Carel, 2008, p. 20). She experienced a body that was no longer delivering; no longer allowing or enabling her to do what she had previously done without thought. Illness in her body was thus inextricably linked with illness in her 'self' – namely her capacity to live her daily life. She described illness as a life-changing and self-changing process, being much more than a biological problem.

In her book, she goes on to consider the work of Merleau-Ponty and his account of the body and perception as 'the seat of personhood' (Carel, 2008, p. 20). He described a proposition that we engage with the world – both perceive and respond to it – through our experience of our body. Multiple elements of our body are involved in sensing the world. These perceptions are then centrally unified to produce a coherent account. For example, my sensation of drinking a cup of tea relies on my perceptions of holding a cup, of something fluid entering my mouth, of that tasting of something I recognise as tea, and perhaps of my awareness of having made/been given that tea before. All these sensations are brought together into an awareness that I am drinking a cup of tea: an awareness that may be subconscious, perhaps until I spill the hot tea in my lap.

If we disrupt the physical body, we therefore disrupt our engagement with and perceptions of the world around us. Carel thus proposes that the disruptive effect of illness reveals the self to be something she describes as 'embodied consciousness'. She proposes that we all have an objective or biological body (the physical entity that is drinking the tea) and a subjective, lived body that is embodied consciousness (the element of me that is, or isn't, aware that my physical body is drinking the tea). Illness changes the way that the biological body interacts with its environment and therefore impacts on our embodied consciousness (our self). In Carel's case, she has a progressive illness affecting her lungs, which limits her breathing and so makes many even simple everyday tasks difficult. Effortless tasks are no longer effortless; automatic things can no longer be assumed; unconscious things are made conscious. The effect of the disruption to the physical body from disease is experienced as a disruption to the subjective body that is embodied consciousness. Carel her*self* feels *ill*.

Carel's understanding of how we respond to an experience of illness is informed by the work of another philosopher, Heidegger. He characterised the essence of the human experience as 'being able to be' (Carel, 2008, p. 66). To be human means being able to respond and adapt to a changing world. Carel thus proposes that the experience of *illness* is a trigger for the *self* to adapt and respond to enable daily life to continue. She recognises adaptability as a highly personal and creative response to disruption of the embodied self.

This philosophical account of illness and the self is mirrored within the sociological accounts of the biographical impact of illness. Carel's own experience of the disruptive account of illness maps to Bury's account of biographical disruption (Bury, 2004). Her description of disruption stimulating adaptation can also be seen in the accounts of biographical reconstruction, reinforcement and flow described by Williams (1984), Carricaburu and Pierret (1995) and Faircloth *et al.* (2004). Collectively this body of literature supports Carel's proposed concept of *creative capacity* as the capacity of the self (embodied consciousness) to respond to adversity, including illness.

For me, there were two aspects of Carel's approach that both distinguished them from other accounts and offered utility for the generalist health practitioner. First, her concept looks to describe not an absolute state of the self, but rather a flexible view of the self that is focused on agency and process. This offers an account of something to explore, understand and interpret in the clinical context rather than an additional 'status to measure' – a view in keeping with the generalist vision of whole person medical care (Launer, 2002; RCGP, 2012; Reeve, 2010). Second, in focusing on ability (and potential) over deficiency, she offered a view of the self that opens options for clinical intervention. My work since reading Carel's account has been to critically explore whether and how such intervention might be possible.

Describing the work of the Creative Self

Emerging from these ideas is a view of an active self, living and responding to daily life. Illness is a potential threat to the continuity, the flow of daily life – something that the self must respond to. Many have written about the work of illness from the perspective of the ill person (Bury, 1984; Corbin and Strauss, 1985; Faircloth *et al.*, 2004). My interest is still to understand the implications for the practising physician – to understand what my role may be in this self-work. I want to understand the potential for health care professionals to either support or undermine this work of daily living with illness. Two research studies helped me in this task.

Exploring the Creative Self in the context of terminal illness

The first was my PhD – an in-depth exploration of nineteen stories told by people living with terminal cancer. I interviewed eight men and 11 women.

Everyone completed a depression risk tool before the interview (the Edinburgh Depression Scale), from which 11 people were identified as being at high risk of biomedically defined depression. At the outset, my intention was to focus on understanding distress or depression. The ideas I have outlined shifted my gaze to looking at the active and creative work of *living* with a terminal diagnosis. During the interviews, I explored peoples' experiences of distress in the context of their on-going work of daily living.

Three different stories emerged from these interviews (Reeve *et al.*, 2010). Most people described maintaining a flow of daily life (biographical flow) – albeit a flow of varying degrees of turbulence. Some revealed episodes of 'biographical fracture' – when the disruptive effects of illness overwhelmed their capacity to keep going, meaning they needed external help to restore balance. One account revealed a story of a terminal diagnosis unlocking prior constraints, so creating a 'biographical shift' – where the flow of daily living, in terms of supporting things that matter to me, had been enhanced (Reeve, 2006).

To understand and explain these difference experiences, I focused on peoples' description of the work that they were doing at these times. Everyone spoke of the disruptive impact of their illness: of feeling 'let down' by their bodies, as well as the practical disruption to their everyday roles and activities. Maintaining day to day living – including adapting to the changes associated with illness and treatment – became harder. People spoke of the challenge to their self-identity – their sense of themselves as a father or wife, as the person who helped others rather than needing help (Reeve, 2006). All of which was experienced as threats to the things that mattered most to them (their 'core self'); leading to distress – periods of anger, upset, questioning and despair.

Yet although the flow of daily living became more turbulent, these stories also revealed that people could maintain continuity through balancing the effect of threats with resources that brought support and comfort (Figure 7.2). For most people, most of the time, this was described as emotional support – achieved through 'releasing' negative emotions (e.g. crying, physical activity) and/or finding opportunities to do things that generated positive emotions (doing activities they enjoyed, spending time alone or with others, allowing themselves to be cared for). Some also spoke of the importance of making sense of what was happening – of being able to find or construct meaning out of events, which in turn offered emotional support and relief. Meaning was constructed through shared reflections undertaken with family members and friends, but also with health professionals. One participant described the comfort she felt when her doctor told her that she was suffering from depression. The diagnosis gave her an understanding of her distress that helped her deal with the disruption. For others, such diagnoses were unhelpful. Mary spoke of her effort to make sense of what was happening to her:

> 'I accept [the way I feel] and I try to find an answer for myself. And deal with it.... I ask myself questions and if the answer is not what I'm looking for then it just brings on a little bit of depression doesn't it?'

Mary viewed her 'depression' as a normal and necessary part of her coping (Reeve, 2006). At the time of her interview, she also met medical diagnostic criteria for depression. Yet she strongly rejected a medical understanding of her distress and instead expected health professionals to support her proactive approach to managing things her way. Indeed she described the potential for harm from attempts to medicalise what she understood as a 'productive depression' (Gut, 1989).

By focusing my attention on understanding the work of daily living with terminal illness, I started to recognise some key ideas. At the heart of these accounts was a 'core self' – the things that mattered most to people. This core self could be threatened by the impact of illness, with associated distress creating turbulence in the flow of daily living. But 'threats' could be balanced by 'resources' – both in the form of emotional supports, and narrative or cognitive supports that helped people make sense of events. Often threats acted as a stimulus for action, mirroring Carel's description of adversity as a driver for creativity. I summarised all these findings within my account of the Self Integrity Model (Figure 7.2).

These findings generated several implications for me as a health professional (Reeve *et al.*, 2009). Most of all, it highlighted the need to interpret illness – in this case, distress – in the context of a distinct individual (self) living their daily life; rather than focusing solely on symptoms of low mood or anxiety. Here, distress is part of an active process of the work to balance the demands on, and resources available for, daily living when faced with illness (terminal cancer). The felt response to adversity – distress – can act as a stimulus for a creative response (Gut, 1989; Carel, 2008). As Mary's account highlights, if health professionals fail to recognise that, and instead offer a biomedical interpretation (a diagnosis of depression), their intervention may act as a threat (rather than the intended resource) in supporting continuity of daily living. The study, and the Self-Integrity model, acts as a reminder for me, and other practising clinicians,

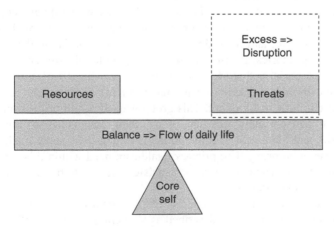

Figure 7.2 The Self Integrity Model.

that when managing presented illness, the key resource can lie within the person sat in front of us. Our job is to seek ways to mobilise, and certainly not diminish that capacity.

Exploring the Creative Self in the context of chronic disease

I started by outlining Carel's (2008) concept of the essential creative capacity of human beings to respond to life, including the adversity of illness. I have described my account of the individual work involved in supporting this creative capacity – to balance threats to the core self with resources, to support maintenance of biographical flow. I have presented data that supports me in thinking differently about my clinical practice – for example, in recognising distress as a potentially productive emotion (Gut, 1989). All of which is helpful in thinking about my clinical practice with patients who are terminally ill. My next question was to consider whether and how these ideas applied in other contexts. I turned my attention to one of the greatest challenges facing today's primary care community – addressing the needs of people living with multiple long term conditions.

The Creative Capacity study aimed to explore whether the principles described within Carel's work and the Self-Integrity model offered useful insights into supporting people living with multimorbidity. Lucy Cooper and I worked together on this project, seeking to understand more about what supported or inhibited individual creative capacity and so comment on the implications for health care practice. We followed 24 people living with long term conditions for a year. In a series of interviews over that time, we explored how people were – or weren't – able to maintain daily living; including the factors which helped or hindered in their daily work. We found that people's stories fitted into one of three patterns of illness experience – which we described as Resilient, Vulnerable and Disconnected. By comparing similarities and differences between these illness stories (Box 7.1), we gained further insights into our understanding of the Creative Self (Reeve and Cooper, 2016).

The first group of stories we described as Resilient. These were told by people who revealed being able to balance illness related demands and threats with the resources available to them; and in so doing, maintain a flow of day to day life. In their 'life for living' stories, people focused mainly on the day-to-day activities of their personal, social and work contexts. Illness accounts (stories of both the impact of their chronic diseases and its management) were largely in the background – present but not dominant. This group wanted health professionals to ideally support, and certainly not undermine, their own (self) efforts to manage their health and illness for example in terms of decisions about medication use and disease monitoring. The primary healthcare need within this group was for individual creative capacity, and its associated actions, to be recognised and valued by health professionals.

Stories in the second group pointed to a risk of significant illness-related disruption to daily living. This group we described as Vulnerable. Narratives in this group were turbulent. For these individuals, illness was making their life difficult and their creative capacity was at risk of being overwhelmed. Daily life continued, but unlike the Resilient group, there was little suggestion that people had been able to integrate illness or its medical management into their daily routines. People revealed being ground down by the work of living with chronic illness. Illness narratives were very much foreground in these interviews, pushing stories of daily living into the background. The healthcare need revealed by these accounts was for health services to address the burden of both illness and treatment – to tailor care to focus on addressing the impact of chronic illness on the work of daily living rather than the management of disease(s).

The third group revealed stories of Disconnect. These were individuals overwhelmed by life events that included, but were not exclusively, disease and illness. In this group, the primary narrative was one of exhaustion – lacking any energy to think about or manage the chronic condition described by medical care. Creative capacity was overwhelmed; peoples' narratives were 'stuck'; biographies were disrupted. These peoples' health needs were revealed as the need to have their exhaustion acknowledged and addressed before attending to any other agenda.

I have described the Creative Self as the capacity of all human beings to live their own life, changing and progressing in response to internal and external stimuli. The narratives from this second study suggested that capacity may differ between individuals, and over time (Reeve and Cooper, 2016). Our analysis sought to explain the differential 'success' in maintaining daily living described by the three groups to offer insights into the nature of that creativity. We identified four factors that appeared to be important in explaining creative capacity in relation to chronic illness (Box 7.1).

People described the importance of things that offered stability in a changing world – what we described as Anchors. These were the core values, the things that mattered most to individuals – things that *felt* important. People actively worked to maintain and protect these Anchors. Next was an active process of Making Sense of experiences of illness, health and healthcare. Here people revealed the work of fitting an illness narrative into a story of daily life and core values. The third element we described as Partnership – the opportunity to 'share the load' of the work of illness, health care with and other burdens with others including health care professionals as well as family and friends. The final element was described by an absence of, or Avoiding Excess Burden. This was commonly an active process of negotiating compromise to make workload manageable.

The Creative Capacity study led me to develop and expand my emerging thoughts about the Creative Self. My next goal was to consider if I could pull all these ideas together to offer new insights for practice.

Revealing the Creative Self

I started this chapter wanting to understand how I as a clinician might better understand, and so work with, the self who is ill. Dowrick's (2004) outline of a

Box 7.1 Understanding creative capacity – relating illness narratives to explanatory factors

RESILIENCE: The case of John

John was a retired salesman, husband and father who was an active member of local community groups. He had been diagnosed with type 2 diabetes after he developed severe foot problems – the consequence of nerve damage caused by his diabetes. When interviewed, he was living with a number of disabilities related to this condition.

For John, his *anchors* were his family and his community work. He *made sense* of his diabetes in the context of its potential impact on his daily living, which determined how he prioritised different aspects of his care. He did this in *partnership* with his clinical team (notably his GP) – negotiating compromises in the package of care for his diabetes to *avoid any excess burden* impeding his daily living.

John's story revealed an account of a relatively smooth flow of daily life (albeit supported by steady ongoing work 'under the surface'). In the foreground was his account of his life as a father, husband and community member. The medical story of diabetes and its treatment was present, but in the background.

VULNERABLE: Sue and George

Sue was also living with type 2 diabetes, but her story was dominated by repeated attempts to improve control of her disease through the use of an insulin pump, and advanced carbohydrate management schemes. Each revision to her management failed to meet the expectations of Sue, her medical team, or both; resulting in repeated searches for further technical solutions. Sue was a wife and mother but her interview narrative was dominated by an account of her medical problems and management with very little time spent on her daily living. She clearly described working in *partnership*, predominantly with professionals. She had, until that point, *avoided being overwhelmed by an excessive* burden that prevented her from continuing daily living. However, her *anchors* seemed to have been diverted to a focus on medical priorities, with her *sense making* revolving around glycaemic control. Meaning that her illness narrative was very much in the foreground, with any other story of Sue having been pushed to the background.

George, another interviewee who fitted in to this Vulnerable group, similarly described, 'I am the way I am because of the tablets … I need them to stop disaster'. Both Sue and George recognised medical care, rather than themselves, as the lead partner in managing their health.

DISCONNECTED: Fred and Mary

Fred was a single man in his 40s who described feeling stuck – prevented from doing anything by his chronic pain as well as complex set of social circumstances. He struggled to describe any *sense of* meaning in what was happening to him, and could see no way forward from his current position. He felt *overwhelmed by the burden* of circumstances and ill health, with a lack of any *meaningful partnership* that might help change things.

Another participant in this group, Mary, simply said, 'I have got no life'. People in this group struggled to describe a day to day existence, but also spoke little about their health and illness. Neither illness or biographical narratives were foreground.

curious, engaged and imaginative self, and Carel's (2008) description of a creative response to the adversity of illness offered me a 'lens' through which to
observe peoples' experiences of living with, responding and adapting to chronic
illness. The emerging accounts offered insights into a creative process of
responding and adapting to the potentially disruptive impact of illness. By
reflecting on all this work, I have been able to develop and refine my initial
account of the Creative Self (Figure 7.1); describing how self-agency – the reali-
sation of the Creative Self in responding to illness – depends on the interplay of
five core elements. These five are the Creative Self, the Work of Everyday Life,
the (Im)Balance between Resources and Demands, the presence/absence of stabilising effects of Anchors or Ballast, and the Flow of Daily Life. I suggest that
both physician and patient need to be mindful of these elements when understanding and addressing health needs, so that both can work to enhance health as
a resource we need and use for everyday living (Williamson and Carr, 2009).

The Creative Self refers to the innate capacity of all human being to change
and progress in recognition of and response to internal and external stimuli. It
refers to the intellectual, emotional, physical and spiritual essence of the individual self which supports the inherent curiosity, imagination, and desire
(Dowrick 2004) of each individual to make sense of and enact daily life. The
goal for health professionals and patients alike is to optimise the capacity of each
Creative Self – to realise the potential for individuals to respond creatively to
adversity. This understanding of a patient as a Creative Self recognises a 'whole
person' model of medical care (RCGP, 2012), where the goal is to support an
individual self in their work to maintain continuity or flow of everyday living
(Williamson and Carr, 2009; Barry *et al.*, 2001).

Each Creative Self needs the resource(s) to Power the Work of Everyday Life
(Reeve and Cooper, 2016). Everyday tasks range from the necessities of finding
shelter, warmth, food, a place to sleep; the social activities of being with family
and friends; our societal obligations in various forms of activities and work;
through to addressing our personal aspirations, needs and goals – of 'being me'
(Maslow, 2013). Each of these tasks can act to both replenish and diminish the
reserves that we draw on to 'power' the work of daily living. For example, food
can nourish us; but to have food we must earn the money to buy it or manage the
process of growing it. Food is both a resource and a demand on our resources
and reserves. Resources can be enhanced through partnership – whether with
social and/or professional contacts (Reeve and Cooper, 2016; Reeve *et al.*,
2016). We need to understand the self within its social context.

Managing illness, including related healthcare, is just one part of a broader
work schedule for each of us (Corbin and Strauss, 1985; May *et al.*, 2014). Both
the tasks of living with illness, and of managing daily routines, occur in the
context of the Flow of Daily Life. Our external world – whether our immediate
social circle, or a broader societal network – inevitably influences the demands
upon us. For some of my research participants and patients alike, the work of
managing illness takes place on a relatively calm background of wider social
influences. Others were trying to deal with the upheaval of diagnoses whilst also

navigating chaotic social and societal influences, for example living in troubled neighbourhoods. The impact of turbulent external circumstances can both create additional demand on, and work for, individuals; but also diminish access to support and resources.

Our daily task to navigate through calm or choppy seas is made easier or harder by the relative (Im)Balance of Resources and Demands on the Creative Self. Individuals in the Creative Capacity study could carry relatively high levels of illness work when balanced by sufficient resources. For example, John lived with significant disability resulting from his diabetes but had strong social networks providing a counterbalance. By contrast, George (another participant in the same research project) was dealing with fewer medical complications from his diabetes but described feeling overwhelmed by his illness and so completely reliant on medical care. George had access to fewer supportive resources so was at risk of being overwhelmed by a lower level of clinical burden. To understand where illness features within a personal narrative of daily living, we need to understand the full range of work being undertaken (Corbin and Strauss, 1985) and the relative balance of resources available and demands upon the individual.

The importance of meaning and values in managing illness is repeatedly highlighted within my research. These 'things that matter' were demonstrated to offer vital stabilising effects – core values acting as Anchors or Ballast when navigating the potentially turbulent flow of daily living. Perhaps the starkest example of this was revealed in my PhD within Angela's story (Reeve, 2006). Angela was a young woman dying of ovarian cancer, yet the story she told of living with terminal cancer was in many ways less turbulent than her story prior to her cancer diagnosis. She described previously having to prioritise the needs of others over her own – the demands of being a wife, mother, employee. With her cancer diagnosis came permission to re-prioritise around her own needs and values. This anchoring of the work of daily living within things that mattered to her provided a valuable support in managing the day to day effects of chemotherapy, a cancer diagnosis and the knowledge that she had only a few weeks or months left to live.

The nature and significance of Anchors is further illustrated by consideration of situations in which this resource is deficient. Tom is a young man in his thirties who presents with an acute psychotic episode apparently precipitated by drug and alcohol use. Tom's medical notes reveal a chaotic story of recurrent crises and the underlying problem has been diagnosed as a personality disorder. The medical term is complex, but in the context of our current discussions means that Tom has a different set of values (ways of seeing the world) than others in his community. The things that matter to Tom are incongruent with the social world in which he finds himself. Viewed from the perspective of the Creative Self, Tom's Anchors offer little ballast, leaving him vulnerable to the turbulent flow of daily living and so to chaotic travel. Tom's story reminds us that our core values, and the things that matter, need an anchor point: a grounding in wider social norms. Again we must recognise that any concept of the self needs a social and a societal reference.

Perhaps, most of all, my work has highlighted the complexity and variability of these components within fluid stories of individual selves working to maintain daily living in the face of illness. The narrative account described here has been, for me, sufficient to support implementation into practice, as I will now describe.

Utilising the Creative Self: implications for clinical practice

At the start of this chapter, I described wanting to better understand the *self* who is *ill* to offer me new insights into clinical practice. I wanted something to help me manage health problems where the disease model alone is insufficient. Can the Creative Self help me think differently in consultations with patients presenting with complex health problems? Let us return to two people I have previously mentioned – John and Heather.

John's story

John was a participant in our creative capacity research study – a retired salesman with a new diagnosis of diabetes. He only found out he had the condition when he developed a problem with his foot. The cause of the problem was discovered to be damage to nerves caused by his diabetes. His mobility was permanently affected by the damage and John was forced to retire from his job.

Faced with significant disruption to his everyday life, John was also struggling to come to terms with his new diagnosis – making sense of what it meant, juggling the multiple medicines he was supposed to take every day, fitting all his NHS appointments in to his diary. John described that he felt all his consultations with health care professionals were characterised by being told he had failed (to meet his diabetic targets), being given more work to do (more pills to take, more tests to complete), and arguments/resistance (about what he should and shouldn't do (e.g. whether he should start taking insulin). At the early stages of John's illness, when the focus was still very much on a medical approach, his story was certainly characterised by turbulence and vulnerability.

In his interview, John described how he was able to work with his GP to shift the conversation instead to one characterised by a focus on the Creative Self. John and his doctor viewed his health-related issues through a new 'lens' which prioritised daily living over diabetic control, and recognised the primary goal of care as to unlock John's creative capacity to respond and adapt to his new daily life. This opened a conversation that considered the resources and demands that John was managing – both in his daily life, and his illness; along with the capacity to power this work. It recognised the anchors and priorities to be supported, rather than challenged, if John was to continue (and extend) his work of daily living. The approach brought new resources into the conversation, beyond a consideration of the medical interventions – notably John's creative capacity along with his network of support and partnerships. It offered new ideas for assessing impact and progress – a shift away from 'failing' targets to identifying opportunities to help John meet his needs for daily living.

The result was a compromise between the actions and outcomes that mattered for John and from a biomedical perspective. With growing awareness of the potential for modern medical care to pose significant treatment burden on some patients, there is growing acknowledgement of the need to find ways to support acceptable compromise between medical and patient perspectives (Kings Fund, 2013; Tinetti and Fried, 2004). The Creative Self offers a framework by which patient and clinician can together explore the benefits and problems associated with different actions and so reach an informed compromise on goals of care.

I started the chapter by describing the beginning of Heather's story. Heather went on to tell me she was frightened that she was suffering from depression. She felt it was the only explanation for why she felt so low, weepy, tired all the time, overwhelmed. When there was really 'no reason' why she should feel like this – she had a job she loved, a home and family who brought her great joy, and no major worries. Other people had been noticing that she 'wasn't herself' and had asked her if she was depressed – suggested she see a doctor, think about getting some tablets. 'There must be something wrong with me,' she said.

Taking a Creative Self approach, my early conversations with Heather focused on her 'work of daily living'. Having explored and acknowledged how she felt, we sought to consider how and why things may have reached this point. Around her, the flow of daily life was quite calm and steady. Heather described that the things that mattered to her were that her family should be safe and well, and that she should be the strong one at the heart of work and home. We explored her Resources and Demands – and noted plenty on both sides. There had been no recent major upset to knock things out of balance, but our conversation revealed a long-standing mismatch between the two. To continue delivering on the things that mattered to her (helping others), Heather had reduced the amount of time she spent, the work she did, on looking after herself – the demands were not being matched by equivalent resource. Heather's capacity to power the work of daily living had been diminishing for some time; but had gone unnoticed – by herself, or by others. Eventually, she had reached a tipping point – a point of complete exhaustion.

The conversation to explore her Creative Self had already become part of the therapeutic process. Our exploration guided the discovery of ways we might address Heather's exhaustion, unlock her Creative Self and so restore daily living. Over time, we negotiated some of the demands that Heather would (temporarily) let go of, and considered how she would access additional resource. As Heather's energy levels restored and she was able to re-start daily living, we worked in partnership to examine the effect of changes and identify or create new ideas for resources. With time, my role diminished and Heather was once again leading, powering the work of her daily life. When new challenges arose (changes at home and work), the flow of daily life became more turbulent again. This time, Heather could respond creatively, and in a different way to the one she had done previously. All without a biomedical diagnosis, or medication. The key therapeutic intervention was unlocking Heather's Creative Self.

Why the Creative Self matters

My research provides both empirical and theoretical support for ideas and concepts that are 'deeply known' to practising GPs (Stange, 2009) and other clinicians offering person-centred (Harding *et al.*, 2016) clinical care. Does my thinking add anything new or distinct?

Exploring the literature, we see several accounts of practice that recognise empowering the individual as a primary goal of medical care. Chan *et al.* (2006) describe the use of the Strength-focused and Meaning-oriented Approach to Resilience and Transformation (SMART) approach in helping individuals to deal with acute crises. Resnick *et al.* (2011) recognise the importance of building both psychological and physiological resilience in supporting healthy aging. Similarly, the literature on self-management describes the goal of care being to enable individuals to take control of their own healthcare needs (Sarkar *et al.*, 2006). To date, these areas of work focus predominantly on improving the management of specific health-service defined conditions. By contrast, the Creative Self is intended to offer an overarching framework to support the individual who is ill.

Launer's (2002) work on Narrative Medicine, also grounded in a biographical understanding of illness, draws on the practical wisdom of disciplines such as family therapy to support clinicians in developing therapeutic narratives with their patients. There is certainly overlap between Launer's work and my account of the Creative Self in terms of the implications for interactions with patients in a consultation setting. What the Creative Self offers that is distinctive is a conceptual framework to guide the development of a therapeutic narrative. This additional element addresses an explicit barrier to delivering person-centred medical care identified in my previous research (Reeve *et al.*, 2013b, 2012): namely, professional uncertainty in articulating the tasks of person-centred care and so describing how to recognise – and defend – quality care.

Some clinicians reading this chapter will recognise ideas expressed here as part of their own established forms of practice. However, evidence from my research (Reeve *et al.*, 2013b, 2017), and my own experiences of teaching these ideas to practitioners, reveal that clinicians at multiple career stages feel that these ways of working are threatened by modern health systems. My intention in this chapter is not to propose something radically new or different, but rather to offer a new articulation of ideas. By opening these ideas to reflection and critique I aim to help the practitioner make critical use of these concepts, but also reveal the nature of and reasons for changes in health systems needed to support this approach. It is to this aspect that I now turn in the final section of this chapter.

From individual to collective application

I have described the development of my concept of the Creative Self, and argued for its utility in the self-focused practice of medicine that is generalist health care. I propose that this understanding offers insights to generalist practitioners seeking to learn and enhance their craft. A proposition supported by feedback from trainees and colleagues with whom I have discussed and presented this work.

But does this way of thinking have wider utility in thinking about how we re-design health services? We recognise a need for change to tackle emerging problems that are not addressed by traditional condition-focused medical models (overdiagnosis, treatment burden, problematic polypharmacy, medically unexplained symptoms) but we are unclear how to deliver it. We hope to enhance self-management to address the imbalance between rising demand and limited resource, but are struggling to achieve this in practice.

I now turn to describe two projects in which I have explored the extent to which a view of the Creative Self can help us rethink service design. This work tackles two key challenges for today: managing mild-moderate health care and addressing multimorbidity and problematic polypharmacy. Both projects recognised that to introduce a new self-focused model of care, we had to change both the work of individual clinicians and the organisational context in which they were working.

BounceBack: a flipped model of primary mental health care

Many people will have felt 'down' or 'low' at some point in their lives. When that feeling becomes sustained, people may describe themselves as feeling depressed (in western cultures at least – see Dowrick 2004) and so present to health services. The best way to manage depression remains a topic of considerable debate.

Today's UK health service adopts a biopsychosocial view of managing depression. Guidelines propose that clinicians should assess whether patients presenting with low mood meet diagnostic criteria for the pathological/biological state of depression. They should confirm the severity of depression using a validated tool (e.g. the Patient Health Questionnaire-9) and use the score generated to guide treatment decisions (including self-management, talking therapies or medication). Within this approach, psychosocial influences on mood are recognised to act as both support and barrier to effective treatment. Practitioners are encouraged to address any barriers to compliance with care.

A few years ago, I came across a mental health charity in Merseyside – AiW Wirral – who were using a socio-psycho-bio model of care. Essentially, their 'flipped' approach recognised social and psychological factors as the primary influences on mood. Case workers would work with clients to address these issues first. Only if mood problems persisted did they encourage people to seek medical (biological) help. Through discussion, colleagues at AIW and I recognised this approach as resonating with my emerging view of the Creative Self – recognising and mobilising elements of the Creative Self to improve health and wellbeing. We sat down to develop a model of care that could be integrated into the primary care setting – combining AIW's experience with the theoretical and empirical work I had done. The result was the BounceBack project. We success-fully applied for funding to implement and evaluate BounceBack into a handful of GP practices in Merseyside (Reeve *et al.*, 2016). Our overall goal was to explore if/how we could deliver a self-focused model of mental healthcare.

BounceBack included two elements: a new way of consulting with patients, and a new organisational model of delivery in practice (ibid). The consultation with patients centred on an exploration of daily living, seeking to unlock an assumed inherent creative capacity. The consultation took a biographical, rather than a medical, approach in exploring a story of disruption to daily living and helping patients to recognise and understand the imbalance of psychosocial resources and demands contributing to their experience of distress. The goal of care was to help patients identify opportunities for change, and then support them in implementing them. We developed the Exhaustion Cycle shown in Figure 7.3 as a model to help with this discussion.

The BounceBack research study aimed to assess whether we could implement this way of working in everyday general practice. We used Normalisation Process Theory (May *et al.*, 2015) – a model recognising the work needed to implement new forms of practice into everyday settings – to guide the introduc-tion, supported by a formative evaluation approach. Our experience of develop-ing and implementing the new service highlighted several barriers to 'flipping' from a biopsychosocial approach to the BounceBack model. These included: the need to educate both patients and clinicians about the new ways of working; to offer resources to staff involved in delivery (including training, access to peer

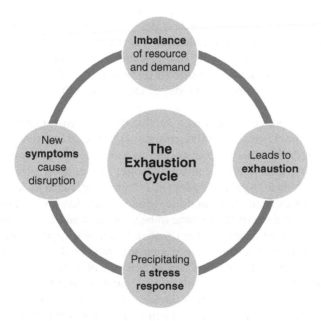

Figure 7.3 The Exhaustion Cycle.

support, and creating headspace); and to recognise the impact of service contractual mechanisms (pay-for-performance) on clinical practice. We used the study findings to revise and refine the BounceBack model – to describe an improved complex intervention that could be rolled out and formally evaluated in other settings (Reeve *et al.*, 2016).

So far, case study evidence from the research project and in continuing practice has demonstrated that patients and professionals like the way of working, which resonates with a generalist approach and patient-centred (self-focused) care. We have seen evidence of the approach supporting the mobilisation of creative capacity – with patients describing moving from feeling overwhelmed (associated with low mood and anxiety) to being able to rebalance daily living. We have also used the approach in managing other complex problems including chronic pain and medically unexplained symptoms (Reeve *et al.*, 2016). Our next goal is a full implementation study with summative evaluation of impact. Aiming to generate the practice-based evidence of whether this model works at scale, and so offers opportunities to redesign primary mental health care around a self-focused model.

Tackling problematic polypharmacy: the complex needs study and PRIME prescribing

We have also applied the principles of the Creative Self to thinking differently about prescribing practice and tackling problematic polypharmacy. The use of multiple medicines in one individual (polypharmacy) is now a common feature of modern medical practice. Whilst recognising the benefits that appropriate polypharmacy has brought to individuals and populations, new concerns are emerging about a phenomenon of problematic polypharmacy (Kings Fund, 2013) – the situation arising when the use of medicines creates a burden on the individual that is greater than the benefit offered (Heaton *et al.*, 2017) Our proposal was that a shift to a self-focused model of care might help address this burden.

The Complex Needs project started as a service development project in a single practice in Liverpool (Reeve and Bancroft, 2014). Our goal was to use the theoretical ideas described in this chapter to help us articulate the professional practice of GPs seeking to deliver person centred care, and so describe a new model of prescribing practice. Again, we adopted a 'flipped' approach in consultations – shifting the focus from managing disease and medication, to managing daily living. The aim of the consultation came to be to understand health, illness and health care need from the context of the Creative Self managing the work of daily living. Decisions about medication use were made based on the potential to support or undermine the activities of the Creative Self, and of daily living.

Nora's story stood out as a key example of the change in approach generated by the application of the Creative Self thinking. Nora was in her 70s. She lived alone and the only recorded health problem in her records was of hypertension for which she was prescribed four antihypertensives. Her blood pressure (BP) was rarely recorded, but always 'off target'. I tried on several occasions to call out to see Nora to discuss her polypharmacy – she was always out. Eventually I managed to speak with her and arrange to call round. Nora told me that she feared seeing doctors because they always told her that her BP was 'wrong' and added more tablets. She didn't take any of the medicines (I emptied bags full out of her cupboards). She understood the principles about BP management, but for her the anxiety of medicines and monitoring outweighed any potential benefit. We, the medical team, had inadvertently become a drain on Nora's capacity for daily living – creating anxiety, and prompting her to 'hide when the doorbell went'. Nora's BP had never been dangerously high – just not meeting a biomedically defined ideal. Through a conversation focused on daily living and Nora's priorities, we agreed not only to stop her tablets, but also to remove the recorded clinical problem of 'hypertension'. The recorded reason for both decisions was that they offered greater risk than benefit to Nora's capacity for daily living.

Nora's case is an example of individually tailored, personalised care; with decision making supported by adopting a 'lens' of the Creative Self focused on a 'life for living'. Her story illustrates that personalised care needs at least an initial investment of resource, offering something above and beyond standardised care (in this case, annual hypertension monitoring). Yet in a resource stretched service, there are practical questions about how we can deliver such an approach at scale; and policy questions about whether it is effective and efficient to do so.

Providing answers to those questions is an area of ongoing research. We ran the Complex Needs project as a service development intervention for a year. During the time, we saw a (small) reduction in levels of prescribing, and highlighted case study examples (like Nora) of reported improved daily living (Reeve and Bancroft, 2014). But we recognised that we would need the resources of a formal research study to answer questions about resources used and wider impact. Since the initial project finished, I have been working with clinical, academic and patient colleagues to develop this self-focused approach into a new complex intervention (PRIME Prescribing) that we can formally evaluate. Work is still in progress, but our initial findings suggest the principles are supported by patients and practitioners (Reeve *et al.*, 2017). I hope that by the time you are reading this chapter, we will have more results to report to you.

I offer the PRIME Prescribing work as an example of applying the principles of the Creative Self to decision making about traditionally biomedically-focused clinical issues such as the decision to use medication. The goal is to bring a self-focused element back into clinical decision making in a transparent and critical way; and in so doing develop the evidence for the interpretive practice (Reeve, 2010) that is the provision of whole-person generalist medical care. Research which leads me into the final section of this chapter – considering how we might roll out a more self-focused approach to health care across the primary care and NHS setting.

Delivering self-focused care at scale: implications for training, practice and service design

The BounceBack project and PRIME Prescribing both describe the implementation of a model of self-focused care to address priority areas for today's primary care health systems. Each recognises a goal to mobilise the inherent capacity of individual patients in becoming part of the solution to their illness experiences, including the need to balance the resources and demands of illness and treatment work. This self-focused, or whole-person, approach to describing and meeting healthcare needs describes the essence of medical generalism (RCGP, 2012). Scaling up the delivery of this approach offers scope to tackle the recognised overemphasis in western health systems on disease-focused (specialist) care – an imbalance suggested to be contributing to the emerging challenges of treatment burden, overdiagnosis and other iatrogenic harm (Tinetti and Fried, 2004; WHO, 2008; RCGP, 2012; May et. al., 2014; Reeve, 2010).

From my own experiences of researching, teaching and clinical practice in this area, I know that many clinicians welcome a shift from a disease-focused to a person-centred, or self-focused, approach to clinical care. However, they also describe clear barriers to delivering this way of working within the constraints of modern healthcare systems and practice (Box 7.2). Scaling up a self-focused approach to understanding and addressing health care needs will require us to tackle these barriers through health systems redesign. The ideas discussed in this chapter start to address the first described barrier related to diagnostic labels. Building on these ideas, I am now working with colleagues to describe and implement the changes needed to address the rest.

Box 7.2 Clinician reported barriers to delivering individually tailored, self-focused clinical care (Reeve et al., 2013b, 2017)

- Current models of service delivery built on the principles of Scientific Bureaucratic Medicine (Harrison et al., 2002) require diagnostic labels to legitimise access to medical care and associated resources ('Depression' is a more legitimate diagnosis than 'Exhausted self').
- Managed health care systems prioritise the tasks of disease diagnosis and management over the expertise of generalist (whole person) interpretation of illness. Clinicians report lacking time and head space for the interpretive practice of self-focused care.
- A perceived lack of training, skills and confidence in individually-tailored care acts as a barrier to care, with clinicians feeling uncertain about producing 'defendable decisions'. Clinicians report a perceived fear in working 'beyond guidelines'.
- Healthcare have failed to adequately protect/develop appropriate systems of monitoring of/learning from self-focused care that is necessary to support the generation of knowledge-in-practice-in-context (Gabbay and le May, 2010) for safe and effective 'beyond guideline' care.

Richard Byng and I are tackling the second barrier – of work prioritisation – in our proposal to redesign primary care services based on a United Model of Generalism (Reeve and Byng, 2017). Our model assigns healthcare need based on the service required to support a self-focused outcome of daily living, where service models are described in terms of the relative contribution of integrated and interpretive care. Our model contrasts with traditional health system models that define need largely by the specialist services available to deliver condition or disease focused care.

Addressing the third barrier related to professional skills and confidence is highlighted within a UK wide review of medical training (Greenway, 2013) which acknowledged a need to train more medical generalists to meet the changing healthcare needs of a twenty-first century population. To achieve this, we must recognise that the complex, intellectual, interpretive task of medical generalism is currently being bypassed by technical systems of guidelines and decision aids designed to support condition-focused clinical decisions (Reeve, 2010; Reeve *et al.*, 2013a). To revitalise generalist care, we need to train clinicians in the scholarly approaches needed to support defendable decision making within an interpretive clinical framework (Reeve, 2010). We must restore (or perhaps establish) understanding of the need for an alternative epistemological framework defining 'trustworthy knowledge' and hence 'best practice' within the primary care context (Schön, 1984; Reeve, 2010b), so that we may also start to address the epistemic injustice discussed by Sally Hull and George Hull in Chapter 1. In doing so, we refute the 'jack of all trades, master of none' view of generalist practice and instead celebrate the intellectual challenge of a clinical discipline grounded in self-focused care.

The academic primary care community is a key partner is delivering this vision. With colleagues from both the Society for Academic Primary Care (www.sapc.ac.uk) and the Royal College of General Practitioners, we are developing work to enhance recognition of, and resources for, GP Scholarship. Recognising that self-focused, person-centred primary care needs expertise, not just evidence (Reeve, Fleming and Bryce, in preparation), we are developing programmes of work to support training in, delivery of, and learning from generalist scholarship. Work which will also support the generation of the knowledge-in-practice-in-context (Gabbay and le May, 2010) needed to address the fourth described barrier in Box 7.2.

Conclusions

In this chapter, I have argued for a model of healthcare that focuses on illness – the health-related disruption to daily living perceived by an individual – rather than disease. My approach is grounded in a view of the Creative Self: recognising the impact of illness on daily living, seeking to mobilise the Creative Self to manage illness, supported (but certainly not undermined) by medicine where appropriate.

Some clinicians, notably generalists, will welcome this approach, and indeed recognise it as something they are already doing. Others, with a specialist view, will prefer to stay firmly grounded in a model of care focused on the diagnosis and clinical management of disease. Both approaches are a necessary and integral part of modern medical care. Indeed most clinicians will need to be able to move between the two approaches (to a greater or lesser extent) at different times (Reeve and Byng, 2017, pp. 292–3).

To strengthen the generalist, self-focused, approach will need changes in the way we train clinicians and organise health care. Changes which may help to revitalise the profession of General Practice – where many practitioners struggle to deliver a complex and demanding workload whilst being viewed simply as 'jack of all trades' technicians. And also help revitalise a health system that is struggling to deal with emerging problems created by an over-focus on disease management, rather than whole person care. The changes needed will require academic input to support them: both in supporting development of the interpretive expertise to find new models of defendable decisions, and in generating the practice-based evidence of good and effective models of care. All of which offers a vision of a new paradigm for health systems. With authors arguing that we are reaching the end of the useful lifetime of the chronic disease model of health care, perhaps we are now ready to move to a self-focused model (Figure 7.4).

In a discussion of urban planning, Fred Kent (2005) argued that 'if you plan cities for cars and traffic, you get cars and traffic. If you plan for people and places, you get people and places'. Perhaps we need to acknowledge the same within health systems and consider whether a change to planning for healthy selves might help us achieve healthy selves. I offer the account of the Creative Self in this chapter as a starting point in that conversation.

Key learning points

1   The Creative Self offers the generalist physician a framework by which to understand, interpret and manage whole person illness.
2   The framework describes five core elements to consider when working with an ill self: the potential innate agency of the Creative Self, navigating the flow of daily living, the resources available to power the work of daily living, the significance of (imbalance) in resources and demands, with the presence/absence of the stabilising effects of anchors or ballast all interacting to support or undermine the work of daily living.

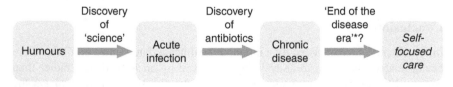

Figure 7.4 Paradigm shifts in health care: describing our changing understanding of the causes of ill health.

Note
* Tinetti and Fried, 2004.

3   Using this framework offers new insights for whole-person-centred generalist practice in the management of complex illness problems including mental health and long term illness.
4   The framework highlights the importance of professional expertise in the skills of interpretive practice to support the development and application of individually tailored management plans to address individual illness.
5   Application of the Creative Self approach into practice highlights the professional and academic work still to be done to critically examine and develop these ideas through practice and research.
6   Work which may, in turn, support the potential for a paradigm shift to a redesigned, self-focused system of health care.

References

Barry, C.A., Stevenson, F.A., Britten, N., Barber, N. and Bradley, C.P. 2001. Giving voice to the lifeworld. More humane, more effective health care? A qualitative study of doctor-patient communication in general practice. *Social Science and Medicine*, 53 (4): 487–505.

Bury, M. 1982. Chronic illness as Biographical Disruption. *Sociology of Health & Illness*, 4 (2): 167–82.

Carel, H. 2008. *Illness (the art of living)*. Oxon: Routledge.

Carricaburu, D. and Pierret, J. 1995. From biographical disruption to biographical reinforcement: the case of HIV-positive men. *Sociology of Health & Illness*, 17 (1): 65–88.

Chan, C.L., Chan, T.H. and Ng, S.M. 2006. The Strength-focused and Meaning-oriented Approach to Resilience and Transformation S(MART): a body-mind-spirit approach to trauma management. *Social Work in Health Care*, 43 (2–3): 9–36.

Corbin, J. and Strauss, A. 1985) Managing chronic illness at home: three lines of work. *Qualitative Sociology*, 8 (3): 224–47.

Dowrick, C. 2004. *Beyond depression. A new approach to understanding and management*. Oxford: Oxford University Press.

Faircloth, C.A., Boylstein, C., Rittman, M., Young, M.E. and Gubrium, J. 2004. Sudden illness and biographical flow in narratives of stroke recovery. *Sociology of Health & Illness*, 26 (2): 242–61.

Gabbay, J. and le May, A. 2010. *Practice-based evidence for healthcare: clinical mindliness*. Oxon: Routledge.

Greenway, D. 2013. *Securing the future of excellent patient care*. London: General Medical Council.

Gut, E. 1989. *Productive and unproductive depression. Success or failure of a vital process*. Oxon: Routledge.

Harding, E., Wait, S. and Scrutton, J. 2016. *The state of play in person-centred care*. London: The Health Policy Partnership. Available at: www.healthpolicypartnership. com/wp-content/uploads/State-of-play-in-person-centred-care-12-page-summary-Dec-2015-FINAL-PDF.pdf

Harrison, S., Moran, M. and Wood, B. 2002. Policy emergence and policy convergence: the case of scientific bureaucratic medicine in USA and UK. *British Journal of Politics and International Relations*, 4 (1): 1–24.

164   *J. Reeve*

Heaton, J., Britten, N., Krska, J. and Reeve, J. 2017. Person-centred medicines optimisation policy in England: An agenda for research on polypharmacy. *Primary Health Care Research and Development*, 18 (1): 24–34.

Kent, F. 2005. *Streets are people places*. Available at: www.pps.org/blog/transportation asplace/

Kings Fund. 2013. *Polypharmacy and medicines optimisation. Making it safe and sound.* London: Kings Fund.

Launer, J. 2002. *Narrative based primary care: a practical guide.* Oxon: Radcliffe Medical Press.

Maslow, A.H. 2013. *A Theory of Human Motivation*. Wilder Publications.

May, C.R., Eton, D.T., Boehmer, K., Gallacher, K., Hunt, K., MacDonald, S., Mair, F.S., May, C.S., Montori, V.M., Richardson, A., Rogers, A.E., and Shippee, N. 2014. Rethinking the patient: using Burden of Treatment Theory to understand the changing dynamics of illness. *BMC Health Services Research*, 14: 281.

May, C., Rapley, T., Mair, F.S., Treweek, S., Murray, E., Ballini, L., Macfarlane, A., Girling, M. and Finch, T.L. 2015) *Normalization Process Theory On-line Users' Manual, Toolkit and NoMAD instrument*. Available at: www.normalizationprocess.org/

RCGP 2012. *Medical generalism. Why expertise in whole person medicine matters.* London: Royal College of General Practitioners.

Reeve, J. 2006. *Understanding distress in people with terminal cancer: the role of the General Practitioner.* PhD thesis, Liverpool University.

Reeve, J. 2010. *Interpretive Medicine: supporting generalism in a changing primary care world.* London: Royal College of General Practitioners Occasional Paper Series, 88.

Reeve, J. and Bancroft, R. 2014. Generalist solutions to overprescribing: a joint challenge for clinical and academic primary care. *Primary Health Care Research & Development*, 15 (1): 72–9.

Reeve, J. and Byng, R. 2017. Realising the full potential of primary care: uniting the 'two faces' of generalism. *British Journal of General Practice*, 68: 292–3.

Reeve, J. and Cooper, L. 2016. Rethinking how we understand individual health care needs for people living with Long Term conditions: a qualitative study. *Health and Social Care in the Community*, 24 (1): 27–38.

Reeve, J., Lloyd-Williams, M., Payne, S. and Dowrick, C. 2009. Insights into the impact of clinical encounters gained from personal accounts of living with advanced cancer. *Primary Health Care Research & Development*, 10: 357–67.

Reeve, J., Lloyd-Williams, M., Payne, S. and Dowrick, C. 2010. Revisiting biographical disruption: exploring individual embodied illness experience in people with terminal cancer. *Health*, 14 (2): 1–18.

Reeve, J., Lynch, T., Lloyd-Williams, M. and Payne, S. 2012. From personal challenge to technical fix: the risks of depersonalised care. *Health and Social Care in the Community*, 20 (2): 145–54.

Reeve, J., Cooper, L., Harrington, S., Rosbottom, P. and Watkins, J. 2016. Developing, delivering and evaluating primary mental health care: the co-production of a new complex intervention. *BMC Health Services Research*, 16: 470.

Reeve, J., Fleming, J., Britten, N., Byng, R., Krska, J. and Heaton, J. 2017. Identifying enablers and barriers to individually tailored (expert generalist) prescribing: a survey of English health care professionals. *BMC Family Practice*, in press.

Reeve, J., Blakeman, T., Freeman, G.K., Green, L.A., James, P., Lucassen, P., Martin, C.M., Sturmberg, J.P. and van Weel, C. 2013a. Generalist solutions to complex problems: generating practice-based evidence – the example of managing multi-morbidity. *BMC Family Practice*, 14: 112.

Reeve, J., Dowrick, C., Freeman, G., Gunn, J., Mair, F., May, C., Mercer, S., Palmer, V., Howe, A., Irving, G., Shiner, A. and Watson, J. 2013b. Examining the practice of generalist expertise: a qualitative study identifying constraints and solutions. *Journal of the Royal Society of Medicine Short Reports*, 4 (12): 1–9.

Resnick, B., Gwyther, L. and Roberto, K.A. (eds) 2011. *Resilience in aging. Concepts, research and outcomes.* London: Springer.

Sarkar, U., Fisher, L. and Schillinger, D. 2006. Is self-efficacy associated with diabetes self-management across race/ethnicity and health literacy? *Diabetes Care*, 29 (4): 823–9.

Stange, K. 2009. The generalist approach. *Annals of Family Medicine*, 7 (3): 198–203.

Tinetti, M.E. and Fried, T. 2004. The end of the disease era. *American Journal of Medicine*, 116 (3): 179–85.

Williams, G. 1984. The genesis of chronic illness: narrative reconstruction. *Sociology of Health & Illness*, 6 (2): 175–200.

Williams, S.J. 2000. Chronic illness as biographical disruption or biographical disruption as chronic illness? Reflections on a core concept. *Sociology of Health & Illness*, 22 (1): 40–67.

Williamson, D.L. and Carr, J. 2009. Health as a resource for everyday life: advancing the conceptualisation. *Critical Public Health*, 19 (1): 107–22.

WHO 2008. *Primary care: now more than ever.* Geneva: World Health Organisation.

Epilogue

Christopher Dowrick

Person-centred primary care

Imagine once again that you are a family doctor. You have finally completed your afternoon surgery. You switch off your computer, put your stethoscope away and take a few minutes to reflect on the patients you have seen during the afternoon.

You were in a dilemma with Edith Brown. Should you continue to prescribe her water tablet, which might improve her heart function but at the same time would reduce her independence, especially her ability to leave home and help others by volunteering in her local charity shop? You were not sure whether your 'objective' medical goals, or the guidance you were receiving from your computer, should take advantage over her 'subjective' life goals and your relationship with her. But the important thing was that you were willing and able to see her as a person, to listen to her concerns and take them seriously. You did not leave her in a position of epistemic disadvantage.

You were also troubled about how to approach the problems Fred presented to you. Would taking an epidemiological view, diagnosing and then treating him for depression and pre-diabetes actually help him? Or would that simply add to his sense of humiliation, of being a nuisance, a moral failure as a person or as a parent?

Your irritation with the computer prompting you to ask about your patient's recent smoking history was yet another reminder of the tension you have been experiencing between standard, institutional views of the patient as one of a population, or as an individual with a unique story to tell.

By sitting on your knee, Millie reminded you, dramatically and forcefully, that one of your primary duties is to pay attention to the person in the consulting room with you. And that paying attention to the suffering of another, recognising their uniqueness as an individual person, can be profoundly rewarding for you, as well as for her. Thus was, perhaps, the pivotal moment in your afternoon surgery.

Although the organ we call her brain might well be disintegrating, and although her view of the world is now very different from your own, when talking with Mrs Sayyid you were keenly aware that she undoubtedly retains consciousness and self-awareness. Like Harry, she can share her thoughts and can still find some commonly agreed meanings with you. Like Laura, she is able to express words of affection and love. Her self-hood may be altered, but you are confident that it retains intrinsic value.

Reflecting on whether or not you should have encouraged Ken to follow the latest health guidance for his respiratory problems, you realise you are comfortable in agreeing with him that how much whisky he might wish to drink is much less relevant than his right to choose how to spend the time he has left to him, in ways that make best sense to him and his family. You share his view that his person-hood, his sense of coherence and engagement with the world, are of fundamental importance, and that he has an inalienable right to determine his own future.

And then, you began a conversation with Heather about her work of daily living. You helped her to see that her exhaustion could be a consequence of her resources not matching up to the demands being made upon her, and to think about how changing that balance might unlock her creative capacity and restore the flow of her life.

All in all, you decide, it's been an interesting afternoon. You turn off the lights in your consulting room, and set off for home.

Searching for the self

And then on your way home, you find yourself thinking about your own view of your self. Whatever your background and occupation, we hope that we have encouraged you to consider where you stand on the questions of persons and self-hood that we have been debating throughout these chapters.

You will probably agree that you are a moral agent possessed with human dignity, with intrinsic self-awareness, and that your perceptions and experiences are not simply by-products of a set of physical, material processes.

You will probably expect yourself to behave as a person with certain moral virtues, with sufficient perceptual sensitivity to advocate for and offer testimonial justice to disadvantaged others. However, sometimes you may feel so con-strained by external demands, whether societal or organisational, that all you can do is conform and submit to a set of predetermined expectations.

You may see your self as an embodied, fleshy affair. You may be comfortable with the notion of being a self-interpreting animal, existing within a body which you can observe, experience and manipulate; and which is itself the medium through which you experience the world and its objects. Or you may see your self-hood as performative, dialogic, constructed moment to moment as a collab-orative social affair. You may consider your self to be dynamic, creative and improvisatory, shaped by socio-material contexts. Perhaps you are intrigued by the thought that your experience of coherent self-hood may not be as firmly rooted as it appears, and find you are attracted by notions of self as illusion, or by ideas about multiple selves.

We hope you see merit in the concept of creative capacity, the idea that all human beings including your self have the potential to lead their own lives, changing and progressing in recognition of and response to both internal and external stimuli. We hope you agree that your self has a fundamental sense of coherence, that you are the unique recipient and holder of all subjective experience built up in stories and memories over your lifetime. And we hope you believe that you are an agent with at least some ability to shape and influence your experiences, through your engagement (whether thriving or struggling) with a unique web of human relationships, and with the wider environment in which you find yourself.

Whatever position you take on these issues, we trust that this book has given you sufficient ideas, examples and evidence to convince you of the need to search for a concept of the self, for both doctor and patient, at the heart of person-centred primary care.

Appendix
Transcribing conventions

[	Onset of overlapping speech
]	End of spate of overlapping talk
[[	Speakers start a turn simultaneously
:	Preceding sound is lengthened or drawn-out (more : means greater prolongation
Underlining	Emphasis
(.)	Pause of less than 0.2 seconds
(0.4)	Pause, in tenths of a second
↑↓	Marked rising/falling intonation
>text<	The talk they surround is quicker than the surrounding talk
°°	The talk they surround is quieter than the surrounding talk
.hhh	Inbreath
Hhh	Outbreath
=	No pause between speakers; contiguous utterances
(text)	Unclear fragment of text
(( ))	A non-verbal activity (e.g. **C** = keystroke in this work)
.	Falling tone (not necessarily at the end of a sentence)
?	Rising inflection (not necessarily a question)
CAPITALS	Louder than the surrounding talk
<text>	The talk they surround is slower than the surrounding talk

Glossary

We here provide brief definitions of the main philosophical or political terms used in this book, on the assumption that not all of them will be familiar to our readers. We do not offer definitions of the terms 'person' and 'self', since these are discussed and debated at length throughout the book.

Action failure the inability to perform ordinary or everyday actions in the absence of perceived preventing causes. A concept designed to distinguish the experience of illness from other types of negatively evaluated experience (for example violent assault).

Agency the capacity of individuals to act independently and to make their own free choices; the independent capability or ability to act on one's will.

Category mistake the error of assigning to something a quality or action which can only properly be assigned to things of another category, for example treating abstract concepts such as the mind as though they had a physical location.

Consequentialism the view that, of all the things a person might do at any given moment, the morally right action is the one with the best overall reasonably foreseeable consequences. Whether an act is right or wrong depends only on the results of that act. The more good consequences an act produces, the better or more right is that act.

Deontology an approach to ethics that focuses on the rightness or wrongness of actions themselves, as opposed to the rightness or wrongness of the consequences of those actions (consequentialism, utilitarianism) or the character and habits of the actor (virtue ethics). It is sometimes described as duty- or obligation-based ethics. In this terminology, the action is more important than its consequences.

Determinism the theory that all events, including moral choices, are completely determined by previously existing causes. Determinism is usually understood to preclude free will because it entails that humans cannot act otherwise than they do.

Dialogic the assumption that language and its meaning are never fixed but always dynamic and relational.

Dualism a theory that considers reality to consist of two irreducible elements or modes, for example mind and body.

Essentialism the view that every entity has a set of attributes that are necessary to its identity and function; the doctrine that essence is prior to existence.

Epistemic concerning the origin, nature, methods, and limits of human knowledge; the theory of knowledge.

Existentialism a theory or approach which emphasises the existence of the individual person as a free and responsible agent, determining their own development through acts of their will.

Eudaemonia well-being, human flourishing. Distinct from pleasure (hedonism), it involves the exercise of virtue, and is derived from a life of activity governed by reason.

Gestalt an organised whole that is perceived as other than the sum of its parts.

Hegemonic ruling or dominant in a social or political context.

Hermeneutic concerning interpretation of evidence, including written, verbal and non-verbal forms of communication.

Instrumental serving as a means to an end.

Metaphysics a branch of philosophy exploring the fundamental nature of reality and being; the general study of how things are or can be or must be.

Ontology the study in philosophy of the nature of being, becoming, existence or reality, as well as the basic categories of being and their relations.

Phenomenology the general study of the character of experience; an approach that concentrates on the study of consciousness and the objects of direct experience; the direct investigation and description of phenomena as consciously experienced.

Physicalism the belief that the real world consists simply of the physical world.

Qualia a quality or property as perceived or experienced by a person; individual instances of subjective, conscious experience.

Reductionism the analysis and description of a complex phenomenon in terms of its simple or fundamental constituents.

Testimonial disadvantage when a speaker receives an unfair deficit of credibility from a hearer owing to prejudice on the hearer's part.

Totalitarian exercising control over the freedom, will or thought of others.

Utilitarianism the belief that a morally good action is one that helps the greatest number of people; that the welfare or preferences of the greatest number should be the guiding principle of conduct. Utilitarianism is an example of consequentialism.

Virtue ethics emphasis on an individual's character, habits, acquired dispositions or moral qualities as the key elements of ethical thinking; in contrast to emphasis on the duty to take right actions (deontology), or on the consequences of actions (consequentialism, utilitarianism).

Index

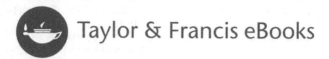

Taylor & Francis eBooks

Helping you to choose the right eBooks for your Library

Add Routledge titles to your library's digital collection today. Taylor and Francis ebooks contains over 50,000 titles in the Humanities, Social Sciences, Behavioural Sciences, Built Environment and Law.

Choose from a range of subject packages or create your own!

Benefits for you

- » Free MARC records
- » COUNTER-compliant usage statistics
- » Flexible purchase and pricing options
- » All titles DRM-free.

Benefits for your user

- » Off-site, anytime access via Athens or referring URL
- » Print or copy pages or chapters
- » Full content search
- » Bookmark, highlight and annotate text
- » Access to thousands of pages of quality research at the click of a button.

REQUEST YOUR **FREE** INSTITUTIONAL TRIAL TODAY

Free Trials Available
We offer free trials to qualifying academic, corporate and government customers.

eCollections – Choose from over 30 subject eCollections, including:

Archaeology	Language Learning
Architecture	Law
Asian Studies	Literature
Business & Management	Media & Communication
Classical Studies	Middle East Studies
Construction	Music
Creative & Media Arts	Philosophy
Criminology & Criminal Justice	Planning
Economics	Politics
Education	Psychology & Mental Health
Energy	Religion
Engineering	Security
English Language & Linguistics	Social Work
Environment & Sustainability	Sociology
Geography	Sport
Health Studies	Theatre & Performance
History	Tourism, Hospitality & Events

For more information, pricing enquiries or to order a free trial, please contact your local sales team:
www.tandfebooks.com/page/sales

 Routledge
Taylor & Francis Group

The home of
Routledge books

www.tandfebooks.com